Health Care UK
Winter 2001

The King's Fund review of health policy

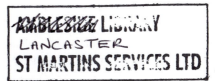

Health Care UK Winter 2001

The King's Fund review of health policy

Edited by John Appleby and Anthony Harrison

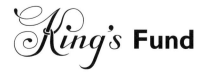

Published by
King's Fund Publishing
11–13 Cavendish Square
London W1G 0AN

© King's Fund 2001

First published 2001

ISBN 1 85717 438 0

A CIP catalogue record for this book is
available from the British Library

Available from:

King's Fund Bookshop
11–13 Cavendish Square
London
W1G 0AN

Tel: 020 7307 2591
Fax: 020 7307 2801

Printed and bound in Great Britain

Cover image: Judah Passow

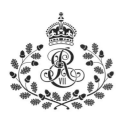

CONTENTS

CONTRIBUTORS

Will Anderson
Project Officer, Public Involvement in PCG/Ts, King's Fund

John Appleby
Director, Health Systems Programme, King's Fund

Penny Banks
Fellow, Health and Social Care Programme, King's Fund

George Blair
Managing Consultant, Shared Solutions Consulting

Sir Cyril Chantler
Senior Associate, King's Fund

Aileen Clarke
*Senior Lecturer in Health Services Research,
London School of Hygiene and Tropical Medicine*

Chris Deeming
Research Officer, Health Systems Programme, King's Fund

Steve Dewar
Research Fellow and Deputy Director, Health Care Policy Programme, King's Fund

Teresa Edmans
Programme Manager, Health and Regeneration, King's Fund

Margaret Edwards
Programme Manager, Primary Care and Older People, King's Fund

Jacky Eyres
Independent Management Consultant

Belinda Finlayson
Research Officer, Health Care Policy Programme, King's Fund

Dominique Florin
Research Fellow, Primary Care Programme, King's Fund

Naomi Fulop
*Director and Senior Lecturer, NCCSDO,
London School of Hygiene and Tropical Medicine*

Pippa Gough
Fellow in Education Leadership Development and Health Care Policy, King's Fund

Anthony Harrison
Senior Fellow, Health Systems Programme, King's Fund

Sandra Meadows
Visiting Fellow in Health Care Policy, King's Fund

Rebecca Rosen
Research Fellow, Primary Care Programme, King's Fund

Ruth Tennant
Programme Officer, Imagine London, King's Fund

Nicholas Timmins
Public Policy Editor, Financial Times

Introduction

John Appleby and Anthony Harrison

The NHS Plan was launched a year and a half ago, and this edition of *Health Care UK* brings together views on the key health care policy issues the Plan addressed. The aim has not (indeed, could not have) been to arrive at an unequivocal judgement about its success or failure, but rather to step back from the detail of the myriad targets the Plan contained to survey some of the broader issues that underlay the document.

In many ways, the NHS Plan was a surprising policy statement – a combination of somewhat laborious and intricate detail about organisational changes, shopping list, exhortation to the NHS workforce, targets (see the appendix to this edition) and restatement of core NHS values. It also set out the Government's view of what was wrong with the NHS – underfunding, a lack of national standards and incentives, staff demarcation problems, a 'siloisation' of services, disempowered patients, over-centralisation and an unsupportive performance improving system. Such a list would not seem to leave much that could be considered right with the NHS.

However, the rather academic Chapter 3 of the Plan, replete with supporting references, set out the positive case for continuing to fund the NHS from general taxation – as opposed to modish calls for a switch to hypothecation, or social insurance, or a straight retreat to a private sector model financed through private insurance. So, at least the NHS is funded in the right way. Indeed, if fairness is the key criterion to judge a funding source, the NHS is one of the fairest systems in the world thanks to a mildly progressive tax system.

And it could be said that one of the complaints about taxation funding – that governments tend to be parsimonious in allocating tax revenues to the NHS – was answered by New Labour when it announced large increases for the Service over the next few years.

The famous pledge – to raise spending to the average of European countries – announced by the Prime Minister in January 2000, was restated in the Plan. From the point of view of the Government, the deal with the NHS was baldly stated in the Prime Minister's foreword: 'We would spend this money if, but only if, we also changed the chronic system failures of the NHS.' 'Money,' he said, 'had to be accompanied by modernisation; investment, by reform.'

To a cynical Whitehall-watcher, this looked like a

typical Treasury deal: the Treasury would never agree to such massive extra public spending without some strong call for change and in particular some idea as to how the money would be used. One view of the Plan was that it was essentially the Department of Health's response to such Treasury demands. If it was, then it fell short on aligning its 'shopping list' priorities with the cost of ensuring that the NHS increased doctors by 10,000, nurses by 20,000, therapists by 6500 …

Nevertheless, the lack of (clinical) staff came top of nearly everyone's list. And compared to many of our European neighbours, the UK NHS does indeed appear to be understaffed. This issue of capacity – as opposed to money – is crucial. **Pippa Gough, Belinda Finlayson, Sandra Meadows, George Blair** and **Sir Cyril Chantler** examine the capacity issue from a number of angles: the extent to which the NHS Plan staffing targets are credible and achievable; possible ways to retain experienced staff; and the way in which existing staff can be used in different ways to effectively increase capacity.

One option for expanding the NHS's capacity is through public–private partnerships. As **Tony Harrison** notes, PPPs can be very broadly defined to take into account all areas where the NHS interacts in some way with the private sector. This will include the buying of operations from the private sector (guided by the 'Concordat') through to private finance initiative deals. While the emphasis so far has been on the input the private sector can make to the NHS, a more open-minded view of public–private relations would also conclude that equal emphasis should be placed on private sector failure and the potential for public intervention.

Chapter 10 of the NHS Plan stated that the NHS would be redesigned to be patient centred. But as **Penny Banks** and colleagues point out, this is certainly not the first time in the history of the Service that this aspiration has been expressed. Within a public service, there is no tidy model for involving patients and the public. But there is scope for going beyond the rather limited vision of the NHS Plan to satisfy growing demands for a more responsive and inclusive NHS.

An important aspect of responsiveness is access to appropriate care at the appropriate time. Of course, the mere existence of a health service largely free at the point of use has been hugely important in reducing barriers to accessing care. However, in ditching financial barriers, the NHS has had to invent new hurdles – waiting lists – in order to cope with the fundamental task of rationing. While waiting lists should perhaps therefore not be seen as a failure of the NHS, but rather a rational response to the inevitable need to ration, the NHS Plan has set targets for reductions in maximum waiting times in primary and secondary care as well as a number of initiatives aimed at improving access more generally. Will it work? And in particular, what impact will the Plan's strategies have on inequalities in the use of health services? **Rebecca Rosen, Dominique Florin, Aileen Clarke** and **Naomi Fulop** ask whether the Plan will meet the challenge.

A key issue for the NHS and ministers is how the Plan will be delivered. The implicit deal – money for change – has put managers under significant pressure to ensure targets are met. But as **Jacky Eyres** and **Steve Dewar** point out, there are real dangers that the conflict between centralisation (ministers want to be sure goals are met) and devolution of responsibility (managers and others want freedom to innovate) – 'constrained innovation' – will pull things apart, ultimately leaving everyone dissatisfied.

In terms of the other side of the deal – the money – an obvious question to ask is where all the new money has gone. **John Appleby, Chris Deeming** and **Tony Harrison** ask the obvious

and find that managers are not only constrained in their innovation due to central controls, but also due to unavoidable financial commitments: there doesn't appear to be much spare cash for local health economies to invest in local initiatives.

There are many more obvious questions to ask: after the NHS Plan, what next? Are we to presume that if the Plan succeeds in its own terms, that's it, no need for any more change?

What if it fails? On what basis is failure to be judged? Indeed, on what basis is success to be judged? There are enormous uncertainties surrounding these questions. In particular, how will the *public* feel about the NHS in the next five years? **Nicholas Timmins** grapples with these questions and concludes that defenders of the traditional values of the NHS may well need to sharpen their arguments.

Patient and public involvement: beyond 'Chapter 10'

Penny Banks

INTRODUCTION

The NHS Plan stated that 'for the first time patients will have a real say in the NHS' and that the NHS would be redesigned to be 'patient centred'. This is not the first time a patient-centred revolution has been promised. In 1989, Margaret Thatcher launched *Working for Patients*, with the claim that 'the patient's needs will always be paramount'. How likely is this latest vision of a patient-centred NHS to be realised and to bring about a fundamental change in relationships between the public and health services?

This chapter will review government policy on patient and public involvement, considering its clarity, coherence with other policies and underlying tensions in implementation. Different King's Fund initiatives and case studies from the field illustrate the issues raised in this analysis and provide some examples of how policy is being interpreted and tensions managed at a local level. Despite the ambiguities of policy and challenges for implementation,

we conclude that there are opportunities to move beyond the limited proposals within Chapter 10 of the NHS Plan towards a more radical understanding of patient and public involvement.

WHAT IS A PATIENT-CENTRED NHS?

The vision of a patient-centred NHS has many possible interpretations. These include an NHS that ensures patients are at the centre of their own treatment, or where patients are involved in discussions about local health services, or where citizens participate in strategic planning to improve the health of populations or local communities. Being 'at the centre' may simply mean people being better informed about all these levels of decision-making within the NHS: alternatively, the vision may be of citizens and patients having real power in decision-making alongside health services or health professionals.

The vision offered by the Government is ambiguous. The Plan primarily focuses on patients and has very little to say about citizen involvement. There is an emphasis on better information provision and customer care through a range of measures, including the new Patient Advocacy and Liaison Service (PALS). Rights of redress, protection for patients through quality monitoring and regulation, and requirements for services to obtain feedback from patients and carers are all within the ambit of good customer care. The emphasis is on patients receiving higher-quality and more-responsive services, but significantly the rules of engagement are set by the NHS.

The debate around PALS and original proposals to offer advocacy from within the NHS provide some pointers to the limitations of this vision of a patient-centred NHS. The concept of a troubleshooter, who is able to feed issues back into the organisation, is welcome, along with more recent proposals[1] for independent support to people making a complaint against the NHS, but advocacy that aims to ensure people can challenge the system and have their say calls for a very different approach. The advocacy movement has long argued the importance of advocates being independent of services, trusted and, most importantly, chosen by the person using advocacy. Good practice in advocacy seeks to empower people to be confident to be their own self-advocates. It is about changing the balance of power where service users have 'more influence over what happens to them'.[2] There is little evidence within current policy of developing partnerships with people that fundamentally alter the balance of power.

Government proposals to 'bring patients and citizens into decision-making at every level' also offer involvement on terms that are set firmly by the NHS. It is yet to be seen whether representation on professional regulatory bodies, the NHS Modernisation Board and other key groups go beyond token participation so that people are genuinely able to set the agenda and influence decisions.

The emphasis on a set of ancillary institutions for involvement is of far more concern as these could work to keep patients, citizens and communities on the margins. These new institutions, including patient forums and recent proposals for local bodies (to be called 'Voice') for every strategic health authority area, may have little meaning to local people and be seen as purely imposed structures, operating on NHS terms. Measures to address other changes needed in the way the NHS works may be sidelined as energy goes into setting up these new structures. This is not only the case within the NHS, but also within the patient movement, which is looking at new ways to support the involvement of people in all these forums, particularly while the demise of Community Health Councils is debated. The more confusing and complicated the structures, the greater the likelihood that people will lose sight of their purpose. Although the Government's commitment to patient and public involvement is made evident through the establishment of new structures, in practice these may do little to bring people's voices to the centre of the NHS.

Policy and how the vision will be achieved is thus far from clear. Government is clearly looking to address the issues of loss of confidence in the NHS, ever-mounting compensation claims and people's changing expectations of public services. But its view of a patient-centred NHS and how this will be achieved, as presented within the Plan and in its recent discussion paper, does not appear to encompass a significant shift of power to individuals and local communities.

COHERENCE WITH POLICY ON PARTNERSHIPS

Other Government policies, however, do offer the possibility of more radical ways forward in patient and public involvement. The Government acknowledges that the NHS alone cannot deliver improved health and health services, and has put partnerships at the heart of delivering improved services.[3] Incentives and sanctions have been put in place to support its partnerships policy. Legal obstacles to joint working between health and social services have been removed, and the Health Act 1999 places a duty of partnership on health authorities and councils. It has been made clear that the NHS is expected to play a full part in the Government's National Strategy for Neighbourhood Renewal.[4] Local strategic partnerships, such as those to implement national service frameworks, are seen as the overarching local framework within which more specific local partnerships can operate. The focus of these local strategic partnerships is to improve the quality of life and delivery of services in a particular locality. Cross-cutting performance indicators have been introduced to support this policy.

If patient and public involvement in the NHS is to be meaningful, it has to be in this context of a major cultural shift in the way services are provided. Managers and practitioners now have to work together across services and systems around a shared purpose. Organisational boundaries and structures are becoming less important than interactions between partners and networks.[5] The challenge for the NHS is to move forward into working in these new ways with local government and voluntary and private sector partners, and at the same time to engage the public as citizens, service users, patients and carers in these new partnerships.

There is every danger, however, that citizens have the least influence in these new partnerships, particularly as different power relationships are played out between local government and the NHS, between statutory and voluntary sectors, and within the NHS acute and primary care sectors.[6,7] At an individual level, patient involvement is threatened where professional rivalries, both within the NHS as well as across medical, nursing and social care, are played out in multidisciplinary teams.

Local partnerships do, however, offer opportunities for better and more meaningful involvement. If patient forums and other mechanisms are properly tied into the local agenda for involving communities, there may be less likelihood of marginalising people's voices and more chance that local people can influence services and the way they work together. Most importantly, there are opportunities to build on local government experience of service user and public involvement, and to ensure people with disabilities and people from all local communities and of all ages are properly included. A two-year project at the King's Fund, which examined the capacity of primary care organisations to improve services for older people, illustrates the importance of partnerships between local agencies in order to engage with older people and have a meaningful dialogue to improve local services. (See case study 1, page 8.)

Open and accountable ways of working are a priority if people are to be properly involved as partnerships develop. The use of flexibilities and other ways of pursuing partnerships offer important opportunities to find a new middle ground between elected members of local authorities and appointed members of primary care trusts. The scrutiny role of local NHS services awarded to local government also opens up new channels for involving local people. Although much will depend on how these new roles for local government are put into practice and whether partnerships are put at risk by fears of takeovers in the formation of care trusts, the pressures towards more open and accountable ways of working offer better conditions for effective public involvement. (See case study 2, page 9.)

Partnership working also turns the spotlight on working cultures within the NHS and relationships with patients and public. The focus of partnership working is on outcomes for people, not patients, which is about people living independent lives in their own homes, with control and choice. This challenges the underlying attitudes within the NHS, where paternalism is still rife. A real culture change is required for two reasons. First, to get shared decision-making into mainstream clinical practice, where people's preferences play a key role in medical decision-making and in disease management.[8] Second, bridges need to be built between the medical and social models of illness and disability. This is particularly crucial as health professionals, managers and clinicians work within multidisciplinary teams, cross-agency commissioning groups and strategic partnership boards. All of this presents a major challenge when much of the medical profession sees itself under threat and so feels disengaged from the whole involvement agenda.[9]

TENSION BETWEEN CENTRAL CONTROL AND LOCAL SOLUTIONS

If partnerships are to be successful, a leadership culture is needed which gives people freedom at the frontline to get on and work creatively. Front-line staff and practitioners are being asked to work outside of traditional boundaries in ways that empower service users and carers. New ways of involving communities and neighbourhoods are being sought to improve health and reduce health inequalities. These changes call for some risk-taking and for finding local solutions with local people, which takes time and creative and flexible approaches. This is graphically illustrated in the case studies of involving local people in the redevelopment of a community hospital and community involvement in regeneration schemes. (See case studies 3 and 4, pages 11 and 15.)

At the same time, government is pushing forward an agenda for change that is giving little time to build the trust and working relationships essential for any successful partnerships, whether between organisations, between different professionals or between the public and local services. Organisational changes within the NHS and proposals for care trusts are threatening the involvement agenda by focusing efforts on making these new organisations work, rather than spending time on engaging local people in addressing local priorities. One carer, commenting on her London borough's action to involve people, remarked 'local consultation seems to have got worse – the main dialogue now seems to be between authorities and central government, not with local people'.

Control from the centre does not sit comfortably with local empowerment of citizens. The ambiguities of government policy and tensions between central control and local action have been analysed elsewhere.[10] A patient-centred NHS, as described by the State and conducted through its prescribed mechanisms, is at the opposite end of the spectrum of open and accountable services where local people genuinely have a voice in local partnerships. The danger is that the rhetoric of involvement is presented in a range of visible structures and the focus is on sorting out these processes rather than delivering changes for local people.

CASE STUDIES

INTRODUCTION

The following four examples from the field, drawn from King's Fund work, illustrate the tensions within government policy on patient and public involvement, as described above, and the pull between meeting nationally determined priorities at the same time as engaging the public in a dialogue about local concerns. The studies underline the importance of the NHS working with partner agencies and show that considerable shifts in attitudes and perceptions are needed on all sides to bring about change.

The two studies of primary care organisations illustrate the challenges and opportunities in forging 'new partnerships with local communities'.[11] Involving local people in the redevelopment of a community hospital highlights the complexities, time and resources needed to engage local communities and go beyond tokenistic consultation. The final example of community involvement in regeneration shows what can be achieved when local people influence decisions about local services and the need for local experimentation.

Case study 1: Primary care organisations engaging with older people

Margaret Edwards

A two-year project at the King's Fund has examined the capacity of primary care organisations (PCOs) to improve services for older people. The research shows that PCOs have started to engage older people in discussions about local services and how these might develop to better meet individual need.[12,13] An examination of this work in various localities demonstrates that, except when they are actually in hospital, older people do not identify themselves as 'patients'. At the point when they are involved in discussions, they may or may not be 'users' of other services such as home care. Their concerns are primarily about the range of services in the community that enable them to live well in their own homes. Their lives are joined up in a way that services and consultation processes rarely are. For example, their experience of using hospital services may be dominated by the intricacies of transport arrangements rather than the quality of clinical care.

The best examples we have seen of involving older people and carers are where one agency, for example the PCG, co-operates with partner agencies to organise activities. This has the advantage of not duplicating work and also demonstrating to participants that the agencies are willing and able to work co-operatively. However, in the localities studied, none had developed a joint strategy for involving older people; the organisations tended to come together at one-off activities. The greatest problems experienced by older people often relate to lack of continuity or integration between different services. An effective dialogue about these concerns requires that a range of agencies are brought together with older people and carers so that realistic solutions can be debated. Single agency forums or consultation exercises will not achieve this.

The impact of age discrimination on the balance of power between older people and professionals needs to be understood in approaches to involving people. The National Service Framework (NSF) for Older People requires the creation of systems to explore user and carer experience, though many of these involve having individual representatives or champions on decision-making forums. The chapter on age discrimination focuses mainly on issues of access to services, though it acknowledges the need to change attitudes and behaviour in communicating with individuals. Our observation of events involving users and professionals in localities revealed underlying assumptions, held by some professionals, that older people lack the intellectual capacity or experience to make valid comments on services. In these discussions, professionals and users commented on how older people's low expectations of services restrict willingness to make negative comments. If genuine dialogue is to take place, then approaches to involvement must take into account the potential effects of discriminatory attitudes and behaviour.

Experience in the field demonstrates how a variety of approaches to involvement will arise depending on the history of local developments. For example, in one locality the PCO has worked closely with a voluntary organisation that has a well-developed network of older people. The PCO has been able to recruit older people from this network to take part in the development of services to frail older people and older people with mental health needs. Where this type of resource has not existed, PCOs have had to rely on more *ad hoc* methods of contacting people, with mixed success in sustaining involvement over the longer term. Most PCOs have set up subgroups to take forward public involvement. These have focused on activities set by the corporate agenda and have in some cases promoted user involvement mechanisms related to primary health care teams. This local approach capitalises on enthusiasm and opportunities: in contrast, central requirements to establish certain systems or comply with performance indicators can stifle this energy.

The major incentive for people to get involved in discussions about services is that they can influence local conditions that will affect them and their families. It is noticeable that user involvement has worked well in smaller localities where people can relate the agency boundaries to their community. National policy has transformed many former PCGs into parts of a larger PCT; our study revealed concerns about this threat to a truly local focus.

Case study 2: Primary care groups: new opportunities for public involvement

Will Anderson

Patient and public involvement is a relatively new challenge for primary care professionals. Although there is a long history of patient participation groups within GP practices, these groups have rarely engaged with strategic issues but have typically focused on fundraising, patient education and the day-to-day operation of the practice. The independence of GPs has also limited the impact of the Government's public involvement policy.

Primary care groups (PCGs) offered a real opportunity for change by providing a new corporate focus for the development of primary care beyond the limitations of isolated GP practice. PCGs have brought new people with new enthusiasm into primary care, particularly officers with experience of public involvement work elsewhere in the NHS and lay members with a brief, albeit poorly defined, for voicing the interests of local people. Above all, PCGs have shifted the focus of primary care development from practice lists to local communities. The public involvement agenda is no longer limited to practice-level patient participation but is now part of the much broader process of partnership across local health economies. There is now scope within primary care contexts to develop health care and health policy in genuine partnership with local people.

The potential for renewed patient and public involvement in primary care is illustrated in the following example from one of six PCGs currently participating in a King's Fund study of public involvement in primary care.

Houndsteeth is a PCG in inner London with a very diverse local population. There are large black and ethnic minority communities and extensive experience of deprivation. There is also a mature voluntary sector and considerable local investment in regeneration projects. In addition, there is a history of health-focused community development work, including some based in primary care.

Although few of the professional members of the PCG had much experience of corporate working, the PCG made an early commitment to working in partnership with the many stakeholders in local health services. The chief executive played a crucial role in ensuring that the PCG looked outwards to the wealth of local community resources as well as inwards to its own problems and concerns. Early on, a Partnerships Manager was appointed, whose role included a public involvement brief.

The PCG convened a small public involvement subgroup, chaired by the lay member, which brought together local enthusiasts including the chief officer of the Community Health Council (CHC), the key officers in the PCG, and local community development workers. This group set out to produce a user and public involvement strategy for the PCG, a process that involved extensive discussion within the group and which sought to capture the breadth of ideas and interests of the members and the range of local activity. It explicitly mapped out the different levels at which the PCG ought to pursue involvement work: supporting user involvement at practice level; building methods of consultation into its own core activities; and working strategically with other local statutory providers.

The development of the strategy was important in defining the scope of the PCG's interests, but it was not used as a plan of action. What the PCG actually undertook was a combination of specific plans, building on existing practice, seizing opportunities, reacting to events and dealing with the torrent of policy from above. This included running local consultation days on the Health Improvement Programme (HImP) priorities, supporting patient-focused needs assessment work in local practices, regular dialogue with the voluntary sector, local consultation on the redevelopment of a health centre, the collation of existing reported evidence of patient and public views, and the initiation of an extensive community consultation on PCT development.

The biggest challenge for the PCG was to ensure that all this activity actually made a difference. Initiatives linked to specific developments, such as the health centre redevelopment and the PCT consultation, had clear targets of influence. But work that was less intimately connected to existing processes of change – such as the consultation events on the HImP priorities – were less likely to find opportunities for impact and change. The PCG itself was inevitably dominated by a centrally determined agenda for change, which left little scope for local influence. Nonetheless, the PCG has demonstrated that primary care professionals can embrace a corporate culture that includes listening systematically to the voices of local people.

Considerable obstacles to the genuine integration of patient and public involvement in primary care remain. Yet the experience of Houndsteeth demonstrates the potential, within the context of a commitment to working in partnership for the health of communities, for bringing community voices into primary care decision-making. Although this process still relies on the presence of key local enthusiasts, their numbers are growing as PCGs open their doors to an ever-wider range of local stakeholders.

Case study 3: Involving local people in the redevelopment of Dulwich Community Hospital

Ruth Tennant

BACKGROUND

King's College Hospital in south-east London is a large acute teaching hospital operating from two sites. Its principal site, in Camberwell, is currently undergoing an £80 million redevelopment to upgrade existing services and bring most acute services on to a single site. As a result, plans are being drawn up to redevelop its second site, in Dulwich, as a community hospital, bringing together a range of intermediate and primary care facilities to support people who do not need to be cared for in an acute setting.[14] This site is likely to fall under the control of Southwark Primary Care Trust, which will come into existence in March 2002.

The hospital will serve a population of around 160,000 people. While parts of the area are affluent, it will also serve areas of extreme deprivation, with high rates of diabetes, stroke and accidents, as well as some of the highest rates of teenage pregnancy and sexually transmitted infections in the country. Big increases in the proportion of the population over the age of 85 are also forecast. Existing rehabilitation and intermediate care services are fragmented and unlikely to meet growing local demand. Measures set out in the NHS Plan to increase the quality and availability of intermediate care are therefore particularly relevant in the area.

The future of the hospital has been the subject of fierce local debate for more than ten years. In 1996, plans put forward by Lambeth, Southwark & Lewisham Health Authority to scale back services provided at Dulwich were contested by Southwark Community Health Council, and a new independent structure was agreed as a way of to take forward future work to develop proposals for the site. An important principal in the new arrangements was that the community should be fully involved in decision-making about the future of the site.

In 2000, with the appointment of a new independent chair, three groups were set up to advise the Dulwich Hospital Project Board on options for the site, including a community involvement planning group.

INVOLVING THE COMMUNITY

A major challenge for the project has been to overcome local cynicism and to find ways to involve marginalised groups in the process. The turnout in both local and national elections is low, indicating a high level of apathy and mistrust of democratic processes. A number of well-organised community groups take an active interest in the future of the hospital, but many of them have a historic distrust of local NHS organisations and fear that the new processes to listen to the community are tokenistic.

Equally, local NHS managers and clinicians, who share with the local people a desire to see a new community hospital for Dulwich, find working with the local community a challenge – staff have found themselves on the receiving end of angry or frustrated groups and individuals. The community is not a coherent entity: different people will have different aspirations for the hospital and the process must arbitrate between these views, ensuring that the most powerful lobbies do not necessary have the most influence and that there is feedback between the community and statutory sector staff.

BRINGING THE TWO SIDES TOGETHER

Building trust between the community and local service providers has been a crucial principle underpinning the redevelopment of the hospital. Work carried out by the King's Fund on behalf of the London Regional Office, looking at Londoners' views on how controversial decisions in health policy should be made,[15] has been used to help develop a shared sense of purpose locally.

Working with different groups of Londoners from across the capital, the King's Fund found that the public place a high premium on early involvement in decision-making processes and on having access to good-quality information to help them to participate on an equal footing with decision-makers. Participants felt that having trust in the people with ultimate responsibility for taking decisions was crucial and that the process of reaching a decision needed to be open and transparent. Equally, there needed to be evidence that the public's voices were being heard and decision-makers needed to explain their decisions fully and publicly.

These findings have been used to inform the way that NHS staff and the local community work together in the Dulwich project. All information about the redevelopment, including information about funding sources, minutes of all meetings and information about local need, is freely available. A 'service matrix' or grid has been developed which sets out the services that members of the community want alongside services that the local trusts, voluntary sector providers and social service department would like to see on the site. This matrix will demonstrate to local people that their views are being considered and will also facilitate dialogue between the community and statutory sector staff about which services will be provided from the site.

REACHING OUT TO THE WIDER COMMUNITY

While the community involvement planning group includes members of a number of local community groups representing local carers, older people, black and ethnic minority groups, local amenities societies as well as both Southwark and Lambeth Community Health Councils, its role is to co-ordinate the involvement of a much wider community living in the catchment area for the hospital.

The group has led a number of initiatives designed to increase the public's awareness of the hospital redevelopment and to give them a chance to add their contributions. A position paper, written in jargon-free language, that sets out the health needs of the local community, initial options for the site and relevant national initiatives, has been widely circulated. A public meeting was held to discuss progress in redeveloping the hospital. Members of the group have worked with a number of existing local groups, including the local area forum, one of six groups set up by Southwark Council to advise them on local policy and to discuss issues of local concern.

Though these initiatives all helped to communicate progress around the hospital redevelopment, it was clear that traditional means of engaging with local people did not necessarily reach some of the more excluded sections of the population. Led by Southwark Community Health Council, five part-time community development workers, funded through contributions from Lambeth, Southwark & Lewisham Health Authority and Neighbourhood Renewal funding, have been recruited to work with traditionally less-vocal groups or groups who might find it more difficult to attend public meetings. Their work has ranged from talking to people on a local travellers' site to working with churches, faith groups and tenants' associations, and groups representing people with chronic diseases.

RESULTS SO FAR

So far, the responses from local people have been wide ranging. Some are sceptical that their views will have any impact. Others are keen to participate but lack the confidence to express their ideas. Some have found it easier to talk about the ethos of the hospital – that it should be a centre for health and well-being as well as providing specific services to people who are ill – rather than the services that are provided on the site. Some are primarily concerned with the physical infrastructure of the building and the environmental impact that redevelopment would have on the local area. Others, particularly people who use the hospital regularly or who suffer chronic illness, have quite specific views about improvements to local services. Many people, particularly older people, support the notion of improving co-ordination of health and social services and increasing local provision of respite care.

BRINGING THESE IDEAS TOGETHER

As well as helping local people to develop their proposals for the site, the community development workers have played a crucial role explaining to groups some of the steps that need to be taken before a final decision can be made about the hospital. This has included talking to groups about different options for paying for the hospital, as well as the planning stages that need to be gone through.

The community development work has been timed to fit closely with formal planning processes. This will allow the community's ideas to be reflected at all stages of the redevelopment. The first stage of this process is to influence the strategic outline case that needs to be approved by the London Regional Office before a more detailed business case for the hospital can be drawn up. A seminar will be held to draw together the different views of community groups, who will be invited to present their ideas to local service providers and architects who have been recruited to develop early options for use of the site. These views will be collated and integrated into the service matrix and will be an important tool for discussing and agreeing a broad service model.

KEY CHALLENGES

The experiences of Dulwich offer some insights into the tensions within the Government's approach to public involvement in the NHS. First, working with local communities, particularly vulnerable or marginalised groups, is both time-consuming and labour intensive. If it is to be properly involved in decision-making, it is important that the public understands the complex nature of the NHS and how it functions, and that time is set aside to allow this to happen. Informed participation requires that people have the information and the support to argue their case on as equal a footing as possible with NHS staff and professionals. Without this, there is the risk that the public will be perceived by professionals as ill equipped to influence local priorities and that public consultation will be largely tokenistic.

Second, limited local flexibility and nationally determined priorities also raise questions about the extent to which there is scope for the community to influence local services. Getting the green light from the Department of Health – whether a scheme is publicly or privately funded – is dependent on making a case not just for how the scheme meets local

needs, but also how it helps meet objectives, priorities and targets as set out in national guidance. In the words of one participant in the Dulwich exercise, 'we can have it as long as it's what the Government says we need'.

COMMENTARY

Involving the community in plans to redevelop Dulwich site has been instructive for both statutory sector staff and members of the community. Both sides have had to make compromises: the amount of time available to work with local people has been constrained by the need to submit proposals quickly and statutory sector staff have diverted time and resources into supporting the community involvement process.

The long-term impact of involving the community will not be evident for some time. It is hoped their involvement will increase local people's pride and sense of local ownership of the hospital, and that it will help make local services more responsive to local need and build a cohesive view of the future of the hospital that is shared by the community and the statutory sector. The project will be working with local universities to evaluate the process of redeveloping the hospital and also the impact it has had on local people. What is clear already is that the community has an important contribution to make in shaping the future of local services and that this is increasingly recognised by staff working in the NHS. The challenge now is to ensure that new proposals designed to increase patient and public involvement in the NHS reflect the complexities of carrying out this work and that staff are given the time, support and resources to do it effectively.

Case study 4: Community involvement and regeneration

Teresa Edmans

Government is committed to involving local people in the planning, development and delivery of regeneration schemes, which, according to ministers, will lead to an increase in local accountability and improved service standards. Existing research suggests that the way in which local people are engaged in regeneration processes can influence whether the health impact is positive or negative and the sustainability of that impact.[16,17]

However, previous experience of community-focused initiatives suggests that there are significant obstacles to increasing community participation. Most communities have had little influence over plans to revitalise their areas or the design and delivery of services. Moreover, the present government's commitment to 'bottom-up' initiatives and local experimentation may be at odds with its strong centralising instinct and continuing insistence on 'zero tolerance of failure'.

The processes of community participation can be challenging:

- communities are likely to identify different priorities to professionals; to be taken seriously, agencies must address the community's priorities
- the process of involvement is unlikely to be meaningful unless the statutory sector changes its culture and its relations with local people
- sustainable regeneration is unlikely unless it creates employment opportunities and community-controlled assets.

In response to these challenges, many regeneration initiatives are adopting participatory approaches as part of the commitment to actively involve the diverse communities in regeneration programmes. Novel forms of engagement are beginning to emerge, with some positive results occurring where local people are increasingly getting involved in their own communities and influencing decisions that affect their lives, and agencies are developing a positive approach to changing institutions to involve the community more in developing services.

Participatory appraisal (PA) is one such approach. It enables a wide cross-section of people to share, enhance and analyse their knowledge, views and opinions of aspects of their lives, environment and conditions. It can also promote working relationships between different agencies and professionals. Application of PA in regeneration schemes, including New Deal for Communities and Sure Start, is increasing. It uses a range of different tools for learning about situations that might arise with people who live in a particular locality. The approach is based on a series of methods to facilitate analysis and discussion of local issues and perceptions, with and by local people. Some of these methods include: participatory mapping, institutional analysis diagrams, historical trend diagrams and matrix scoring of priorities or criteria.

However, PA is much more than just a tool bag of techniques: it involves a major shift in the way in which organisations engage with the community and it requires a commitment to listen carefully to what local people have to say, and to respect the value of local perceptions, issues and priorities. In other words, it has the potential to facilitate institutional change.

EXAMPLE 1: PARTICIPATORY APPRAISAL IN HARINGEY'S SURE START

The PA project was carried out over a five-month period during 2000/01. The aims were to involve community members in identifying problems and issues facing families with children under four years old, and to help identify the availability of and need for local services and facilities. Professionals from the local statutory and voluntary sectors and local residents (including participants from the black and minority ethnic communities) were trained in and carried out the PA. Real changes occurred as a result of the project, including moves to improve the park and leisure facilities in the area, a review of child care provisions in the borough, and the formation of local support groups for parents. The unintended outcome was that, following the appraisal, different initiatives came together to plan further PA work. This will be a joint effort between local parents, the local NDC, the SRB, the community health service and the local Neighbourhood Renewal Fund to ensure that services are developed in line with local needs across agencies.

EXAMPLE 2: COMMUNITY-LED SRB INITIATIVE IN LEWISHAM

This project involved local people in the pre-bid stage of developing a regeneration proposal. A group of local community organisations formed the NX Project and provided training in PA for local people and supported them in carrying out their own research to identify issues, priorities and local solutions. As a result, the local community led a successful SRB6 bid. The work of continuing the involvement of the local communities and building or increasing their capacity to design, develop and deliver regeneration initiatives is ongoing and has led to several other local successes.

COMMENTARY

These two examples show that, while it can lead to sustainable local improvements, community involvement in regeneration requires:

- community participation in identifying priorities
- empowerment of local people by giving them some control over developments and services
- risk-taking and finding local solutions with local people, which takes time and creative and flexible approaches
- resources to ensure that skills are developed so that local people can be actively involved
- commitment to involvement as a continual process rather than a 'one off' to satisfy the bidding process.

However, using approaches such as PA to engage the community is not enough. There needs to be a parallel process of developing statutory and voluntary agencies involved in regeneration to understand the benefits and barriers of community involvement, while at the same time developing their skills to actively engage with the community. Only then will it be possible for the agencies to move beyond consultation and towards active participation of diverse communities.

CONCLUSION

The case studies show there is much to build on and opportunities to work towards a patient-centred NHS beyond the more limited vision within the NHS

Plan. If the Government's recently stated intentions are to be realised – to 'move away from an outdated system of patients being on the outside, towards a new model where the voices of patients, their carers and the public are heard through every level of the Service, acting as a powerful lever for change and improvement'[18] – seven key points need to be addressed:

1. The NHS Plan cannot be delivered by the NHS working alone. Policies on patient and public involvement need to be relevant and suited to the changing nature of the NHS, which has to look beyond its own boundaries to new partnerships with local government and voluntary, private and other organisations.

2. Improving and changing public services requires the involvement of local communities in these partnerships, so local people – not only 'patients' – identify their priorities. Local participation will mean people will look beyond traditional service 'silos' and will connect local services in ways that are meaningful and more likely to make a difference for local citizens.

3. Every member of these partnerships – statutory, voluntary and private organisations – needs to ensure its own organisation works in such a way that involving people is integral to every part of its operation. This involves more than training or raising staff awareness. Systems need to support good practice and reinforce approaches that ensure patients and carers have the information to make their own choices and to challenge without reprisal. For the NHS, this includes changing relationships with individual patients so people have full information to make choices and be properly involved in decision-making about their own treatment, as well as involving patients, public and carers in the planning, development and monitoring of services.

4. There is no one tidy model for public involvement. Local partnerships will need to work together with local people to agree how they would prefer to be involved and influence local services. This will be an ongoing and ever-changing process.

5. Local partnerships must ensure public participation is inclusive. Priority should be given to reaching out to local people – whatever their age, disability or illness, and from all communities – and engaging with them in ways they prefer. Unpaid carers as well as front-line staff need to be included as their experience and expertise provide valuable insights into the quality of local services.

6. Local people will not be effectively involved unless there is an open, honest and transparent debate, where people have a good understanding of the NHS and local services, how the services work together, the resources and who is accountable for final decisions and service delivery. This means decision-making needs to be devolved within a proper democratic framework.

7. Involvement must lead to demonstrable change or at the very least clarity about why action has been delayed or prevented.

There are no easy answers to many of the dilemmas and challenges raised, but the alternative of a paternalistic, largely closed NHS is no longer acceptable to an electorate that wants change. The NHS Plan has opened a useful debate; this now needs to be taken out to local communities, across the Health Service, local government and voluntary sector to shape new approaches and move beyond the limited vision of patient and public involvement within Chapter10.

1   Department of Health. *Involving patients and the public in healthcare: a discussion document*. London: Department of Health, 2001.

2   Thompson C, editor. *Changing the balance – power and people who use services*. London: Community Care Project NCVO, 1991.

3   Department of Health. *Modernising health and social services: national priorities guidance*. London: Department of Health, 1998.

4   Cabinet Office. *National Strategy for Neighbourhood Renewal: a framework for consultation*. London: Cabinet Office, 2000.

5   Henwood M, Hudson B. *Partnership and the NHS Plan: cooperation or coercion? The implications for social care*. Leeds: Nuffield Institute for Health, 2000.

6   Local Government Association. *Partnerships with health: a survey of local authorities. Research briefing two*. London: LGA, 2000.

7   Audit Commission. *The way to go home: rehabilitation and remedial services for older people*. London: Stationery Office, 2000.

8   Merry P, editor. *NHS Confederation Wellards NHS Handbook 2001/02*. Sixteenth Edition; Section 3; Coulter A. *Patients and the NHS*. East Sussex: JMH Publishing Ltd, 2001.

9   Gillam S, Brooks F, editors. *New beginnings: towards patient and public involvement in primary health care*. London: King's Fund, 2001.

10 Hunter D. Managing the NHS. In: Appleby J, Harrison A, editors. *Health Care UK. Winter 2000*. London: King's Fund, 2000: 69–76.

11 Department of Health. *Shifting the balance of power within the NHS: securing delivery*. London: Department of Health, 2001.

12 Edwards M. *Primary care groups and older people: signs of progress*. London: King's Fund, 2000.

13 Edwards M. *Primary care organisations: the pace of change*. London: King's Fund, 2001.

14 See pp 56–62 of this volume.

15 Staley K. *Voices, values and health: involving the public in moral decisions*. London: King's Fund, 2001.

16 Popay J et al. *Regeneration and health: a selected review of research*. London: King's Fund and Nuffield Institute for Health, 2001.

17 Taylor M. *Unleashing the potential: bringing residents to the centre of regeneration*. York: Joseph Rowntree Foundation, 1995.

18 Department of Health. *Involving patients and the public in healthcare. Op. cit.*

Improving access, maintaining fairness: will the NHS Plan meet the challenge?

Rebecca Rosen, Dominique Florin,
Aileen Clarke and Naomi Fulop

INTRODUCTION

The concept of access to NHS care is paradoxical. Launched as a universal service free at the point of delivery, the NHS instantly overcame the access problems of those who could not afford medical care. Yet access has been limited since soon after its inception by long waiting lists for outpatient clinics and inpatient stays. For almost two decades, tabloid newspapers have delivered lurid tales of patients suffering on casualty trolleys, of children being driven round the country looking for intensive care beds and of pensioners living in pain while they wait years for hip operations. Alongside these hospital failures have been growing problems with community services – difficulty getting GP appointments and understaffed community nursing teams contributing to delayed hospital discharges, to name but two.

This cocktail of deficiencies in NHS care is increasingly clustered under the broad title of problems with 'access' to care. Improving access has become a central aim of NHS policy and this goal is evident throughout the NHS Plan. Many of the targets and service developments proposed within the Plan aim to reduce waiting times, increase the provision of staff and services, and make them more convenient for patients. While the initiatives will increase overall access, there is no consideration of whether they will benefit all equally.

This chapter will review the potential impact of the NHS Plan on access to care, with particular reference to its likely impact on inequalities in the use of health services. After exploring and defining the concept of access, *Dominique Florin* considers how proposals in the NHS Plan might affect access to primary care. *Aileen Clarke* and *Naomi Fulop* consider the implications of these proposals for the acute sector. In the final section, *Rebecca Rosen* draws conclusions about what the NHS Plan may be able to deliver and the importance of evaluating the impact of proposed developments on equity.

WHAT DO WE MEAN BY ACCESS?

Access has become an umbrella term for numerous issues about the use and availability of health services. Papers on access vary in their focus, looking at characteristics such as: delays in access and the impact of queuing;[1] service provision and availability;[2] inequalities in the availability and use of services;[3] and the links between access and demand for care.[4] Recent government policy has focused particularly on timeliness and convenience for patients. Other important questions raised in papers on access include those by Florin[5] and the Royal College of General Practitioners.[6]

Access was a key theme in the 1997 White Paper,[7] which made a renewed commitment to the fundamental principle of the NHS offering free access to comprehensive services according to need. While this commitment is reiterated in the NHS Plan, greater emphasis is placed on increasing the patient focus of the NHS and in particular on the provision of 'fast and convenient care'.[8]

In the wake of the Plan, the National Patient Access Team (NPAT) is driving forward a range of organisational changes to improve access (see below), and regional Access Task Forces have been established to co-ordinate other developments. Performance indicators on access developed in response to the Plan are gathered under the title of 'fair access'[9] and include measures of the timeliness and availability of services, age–sex variations in use, and selected data on ethnicity. However, no precise and comprehensive definition of 'fair access' is offered, though the indicators imply that targets for access relate to *who is accessing services* as well as how fast they

are obtained. They highlight the many different dimensions of access that are rarely made explicit. Before considering the impact of current policies, the term will be more fully explored.

THE MANY DIMENSIONS OF ACCESS

The many meanings of access mentioned above illustrate the complexity of the concept in relation to health services and highlight the lack of common understanding of the term. A straightforward definition is difficult to produce,[10] but the key facets of access are identified as follows:

ABSOLUTE AND RELATIVE ACCESS

A key distinction is made between initiatives that seek to increase the overall availability of health services – hereafter referred to *absolute access* – and those that seek to reduce inequalities in access. Given relative differences in the use of services by different groups (distinguished by age, sex, ethnicity, culture, etc.), the latter is referred to as *relative access*.

THE CHARACTERISTICS OF USERS AND OF HEALTH SERVICES THEMSELVES THAT DETERMINE ACCESS

Social, demographic and cultural characteristics of individuals and populations are widely recognised as shaping the use of health services. Thus, age, gender, ethnicity, class, level of education and wealth have all been shown to affect the way people use health services. Likewise, characteristics of the services, including their location, opening hours, who staffs them and how patients are referred into them, are also key determinants of access.

It is often the interface between specific characteristics of a service and characteristics of users that shape access. For example, if female gynaecologists are not available in a district with a large Asian community, use of these services and uptake of cervical screening programmes may be reduced. Access to the service may be physically possible but culturally unacceptable. In a community-based example, access to a primary health centre was shown to be restricted – particularly for older people – by its location at the top of a hill and the absence of a local bus service.[11]

ACCESS TO EFFECTIVE AND APPROPRIATE SERVICES

Developments that increase access to health services will not necessarily improve health. To do so, *clinically effective* services must be offered to a group of patients with *relevant clinical needs*. Furthermore, if these new services are not carefully tailored to the social and cultural needs of local communities, then even if they can be proved to be clinically and cost-effective, they may fail to improve health because of poor uptake.

ACCESS AND DEMAND

The success of efforts to improve access will depend partly on their impact on demand. Initiatives aimed at services with long waiting lists or long waiting times may result in only temporarily improved access if they trigger an increase in demand.

ACCESS AND FAIRNESS

The concept of access – particularly relative access as defined above – is closely linked to the concept of equity and thus to the idea of fairness. Definitions of equity include: equal access regardless of need; equal access for equal need; equal utilisation for equal need; and equal access to health outcomes.[12] These

distinctions are not academic, since many recent service innovations have aimed to improve access through increased availability without necessarily considering their impact on equity in terms of utilisation or provision. Moreover, there will be opportunity costs in terms of health interventions forgone and the relative distribution of benefits obtained and opportunities missed.

ACCESS AND THE NHS PLAN – A UNI-DIMENSIONAL VIEW?

Given the complexity and breadth of the concept of access outlined above, it becomes evident that initiatives in the NHS Plan to improve access to NHS services focus particularly on absolute access – most specifically on timeliness and convenience to patients – with a lesser focus on relative access.

This is not to say, however, that no current policies aim to improve relative access. A further problem with the complexity of 'access terminology' is the difficulty of labelling all relevant policies and developments as initiatives to improve access. Thus, several recent policies that fall into different 'headline' categories may well contribute to improved access.

These include the formation of Health Action Zones[13] and Healthy Living Centres[14] and the requirement for every NHS Region to establish an inequalities task force. And the commitment to look after people 'in the right environment and in the right way'[15] acknowledges – at least by inference – the importance of responding to individual and community beliefs and needs, and providing appropriate, effective care.

The following two sections will consider those parts of the NHS Plan that will most directly contribute to improved access in relation to primary and acute sector care. They will focus particularly on their likely impact on absolute and relative access. The final section will reflect briefly upon the importance of evaluating service developments in order to understand their impact on all relevant dimensions of access.

ACCESS IN PRIMARY CARE – THE NHS PLAN AND BEYOND

In this section we review a raft of current policies and describe recent trends in primary care aimed at improving access. These raise a number of key issues that we discuss on page 25. In addition to the impact of recent policies on absolute and relative access we also consider them in relation to self-care, demand for services and clinical and cost-effectiveness.

It is a legitimate policy aim to improve either absolute or relative access – or indeed both. To this end, it is important to think systematically about what aspect of access is being targeted, about how best to achieve particular access aims and how to monitor the effects of changes to improve access. Clearly health care is a dynamic system, and changes that affect access (whether absolute or relative) at one point can affect other parts of the system. As discussed below, several recent access policies have demonstrated that improving access does not necessarily reduce demand. The impact of access policies in primary care shows that it is overly simplistic to consider access in isolation from other parameters of the primary care system, such as workforce issues, cost-effectiveness and demand management.

Policy is not homogeneous or monolithic, and consideration of access in primary

care extends beyond the NHS Plan. For example, the personal medical service (PMS) pilots described below were launched well before the NHS Plan and have contributed to improved access to primary care. While the Plan contains many new suggestions, since its publication only relatively few of these have been turned into practice. The extent of implementation over the next few years remains to be seen.

'ACCESS POLICIES' IN PRIMARY CARE

The NHS Plan contains a range of different policies and suggestions that may improve both absolute and relative access in primary care. There have also been other recent changes and trends in primary care that are not specifically mentioned in the NHS Plan but which are nevertheless relevant to improving access. These include both professionally driven changes in practice and the results of earlier policy initiatives. Here, the different trends and policies are classified into overlapping categories. These demonstrate that improving access depends on increasing capacity and/or flexibility.[16]

MAJOR NEW PROVISION

Shortly after its election in 1997, and well before the NHS Plan, New Labour initiated two significant new ways for people to access primary care – NHS Direct and walk-in centres. NHS Direct is a nurse telephone advice line that became available in 2000. The aims of the service are to provide 24-hour health advice, to encourage self-care and to reduce demands on other NHS services. Evaluations have shown a largely out-of-hours advice service which is growing in popularity, receives high satisfaction ratings and seems to be safe.[17,18,19] It has proved more difficult to demonstrate either an increase or a decrease in self-care and self-reliance, and little impact has been demonstrated on changed use of A&E and ambulance services. An association, which may or may not be causal, has been noted with a halting in the upward rise in use of GP co-operatives.

However, evaluations have not yet answered a number of other important questions, including effects on equity (relative access). Initially, NHS Direct was offered only in English, but is increasingly available to those whose first language is not English by linking with a telephone interpreter service. Indeed, the NHS Plan has suggested that the service could be used to provide a telephone translation service for patients in face-to-face consultations. At present NHS Direct is used mainly as an out-of-hours service, yet groups with relatively higher use of GP out-of-hours services,[20] including elderly people and those from some ethnic minorities, are currently those least likely to use NHS Direct.[21]

The NHS Plan suggests that NHS Direct should become the single point of access for all out-of-hours contacts. Others have suggested that it could be the gateway for all NHS contacts at any time of day or night.[22] These proposals could reduce equity of access if selected groups are less likely to use the service, and careful monitoring of the characteristics of users will be essential to identify emerging inequity at an early stage.

Walk-in centres were announced by the Prime Minister in April 1999, and 40 such NHS centres are now open, at an initial cost of £31 million.[23] These are mainly nurse-led services open to all-comers, without appointment, seven days a week and until 10 or 11 p.m. The full

evaluation of walk-in centres is not yet complete but early work shows that they provide an open-access service for people with minor ailments, and overlap significantly with services provided in traditional general practice.[24]

The major rationale for walk-in centres is convenience, particularly for workers. This is reflected in the extension of opening beyond normal working hours and their siting in places such as airports and shopping centres. However, Mountford and Rosen[25] found that their ability to fill gaps in local primary care services and respond to local needs has been compromised by tight central control over the range of services that every centre must offer, limiting the resources available for locally driven development.

At present little is known about the overall impact of walk-in centres in the UK, though, as a relatively small-scale development, they seem unlikely to significantly influence relative or absolute access to primary care.

TECHNOLOGICAL INNOVATIONS

NHS Direct and walk-in centres draw upon technological developments to support primary care – specifically the use of telephone consultations and computerised guidelines. The NHS Plan makes other suggestions based on new technologies for communication between patients and health professionals. These include the use of e-mail consultations (so far a few enthusiasts have set these up) and the use of digital TV to give patients advice in their own homes. Expansion of existing telemedicine technologies that use real-time video cameras to communicate information between patient and clinician may also occur. This could be used to facilitate consultations with consultants where geographical access is a problem (e.g. in the Scottish Highlands) or for hard-pressed specialties such as dermatology in order to increase throughput by cutting down face-to-face consultations.

However, telemedicine is not yet widespread and most telemedical practice to date has provided new forms of access to secondary care. Furthermore, little high-quality research has been conducted into the cost-effectiveness of telemedicine[26] and little is know about relative use by different groups. It is intuitively possible that the use of computers and information technology may be difficult for some groups, particularly those without computers or the skills to use them, though equally it may be beneficial to others. This question of relative access should be investigated as part of the evaluation of such developments.

INCREASED ACCESS THROUGH INCREASED FLEXIBILITY – PROFESSIONAL ROLE CHANGES AND NEW WAYS OF WORKING

Integral to many attempts to improve access has been the elision and expansion of roles of members of the primary health care team, particularly doctors and nurses. We have seen the development of nurse practitioners, nurse triage, nurses taking on traditional medical roles, and GPs and nurses taking on management functions and complex chronic disease care. The NHS Plan restates the trend for expanded nurse roles, particularly into prescribing. The Plan also suggests expansion of the pharmacist role, specifically as a way of reducing demand on GP surgeries, for example by taking on the responsibility for repeat prescribing.

With respect to improving access, the expansion of professionals' roles is a way of increasing flexibility without necessarily increasing staff numbers. The effect on relative access is largely unknown.

A further pledge in the Plan is to give all patients access to a GP within 48 hours by 2004. To achieve this target, systems for re-organising primary care to achieve 'advanced access' are being disseminated through the National Primary Care Collaborative.[27] The Collaborative supports primary health care teams in reorganising practice work to 'do today's work today'. Practices are encouraged to change the ways they work, including increasing use of telephone triage and consultations, more nurse consultations, and offering appointments only at short notice to reduce non-attenders. The collaborative demonstrates that significant changes can be achieved without increasing staff numbers, though no formal evaluation has been produced and anecdotal reports from GPs have been mixed.

INCREASED ACCESS THROUGH INCREASED CAPACITY

In international terms, the UK is relatively 'under-doctored' and there are currently 17,000 nurse vacancies in an NHS workforce of 300,000. The NHS Plan promises an increase of 20,000 nurses by 2004, but this figure is disputed by the Royal College of Nurses since it does not refer to whole-time-equivalent staff.

There is also an imminent crisis in GP numbers as the large number of doctors recruited from overseas in the 1960s are now reaching retirement. This is aggravated by the fact that the popularity of general practice with newly qualified doctors fell during the 1990s.[28] The NHS Plan pledges 2000 extra GPs, which professional bodies claim is insufficient to cover forthcoming retirements *and* meet other targets such as 48-hour access. With regard to relative access, the Plan also pledges to improve the distribution of GPs nationally to reduce current inequalities in distribution that result in up to 50 per cent more GPs in relatively less deprived areas.

ORGANISATIONAL CHANGE IN PRIMARY CARE

A number of organisational changes are also relevant to access in primary care. Further expansion of the PMS scheme[29] was announced in the NHS Plan, offering one way in which relative access can be improved. PMS has helped to facilitate the provision of primary care services in areas that have been under-provided for many years and to groups with relatively poorer access, such as refugees and the homeless. PMS also addresses the recruitment and retention problem among GPs by offering a salaried alternative to those who are unwilling to opt for partnership. However, it appears that the recent launch of fourth wave PMS has been less popular with GPs than was predicted.[30]

The now relatively well-established development of GP co-operatives to provide out-of-hours care continues. This development has fulfilled a dual role of decreasing the out-of-hours burden on GPs while also improving access to high-quality out-of-hours care to patients. A New Labour construction is that out-of-hours care is about care at convenient times, but research confirms an important equity aspect. Both the National Patient Survey and other work have shown that traditionally disadvantaged groups – those from deprived areas, elderly people

and those from ethnic minorities – are more likely to use out-of-hours care.[31,32] The reasons for this are not fully understood but may reflect difficulty in accessing care in 'normal' hours. Furthermore, some areas of clinical care routinely require care out-of-hours – such as palliative care or mental health services.[33,34]

Disentangling these different access needs is complicated. Making NHS Direct the single triage point out-of-hours may be one solution – provided evidence does not emerge of growing inequalities in access to and use of the services. However, better access to care within hours is also required.

WHAT ARE THE UNDERLYING ISSUES?

RELATIVE AND ABSOLUTE ACCESS

The initiatives described above will affect absolute and relative access to primary care to different extents. Whether they will address each form of access sufficiently is not clear. With regard to absolute access, the major innovations of both NHS Direct and walk-in centres increase overall provision, and NHS Direct stands to fundamentally change the way we gain access to health care. In contrast to this major change, the relatively modest proposed increase in the number of new doctors and nurses seems unlikely to make much impact in the key area of workforce under-supply. System flexibilities arising from innovations such as changes in nurses' roles will help in part, but again it is not yet clear whether they will make a sizeable enough impact.

While the headline primary care policies of NHS Direct, walk-in centres and increased staff numbers are about absolute access, other policies beyond the NHS Plan may affect relative access more.

These include the expansion of PMS, the use of NHS Direct as a translation service, and initiatives relating to Health Action Zones and Healthy Living Centres. Again, whether they will address inequity sufficiently is not clear. One criticism of the NHS Plan is that it 'favours' absolute access over relative access. While there is clearly a consumerist angle that reflects the former, systematic evaluation of the relative access effects of the totality of planned policies is an important first step to improving relative access. This would make it possible to prioritise modifications to NHS Direct or the organisation of walk-in centres to encourage greater use by disadvantaged groups.

SELF-CARE, APPROPRIATENESS AND DEMAND MANAGEMENT

The NHS Plan is keen to promote self-care, presumably in order to reduce demand in relation to minor ailments and improve access for people with greater needs. While easy access to NHS Direct might appear to support this goal, this concept of self-care is not a simple one.

In one sense, phoning an NHS-funded helpline or consulting a nurse at a walk-in centre is no more self-care than is consulting a GP. There have been claims from the medical profession that increased access will decrease self-care and increase dependency and demand, and there is a possibility that patients may choose to use NHS Direct or walk-in centres repeatedly and possibly 'inappropriately'. Professional constructions of appropriateness do not readily tally with lay understandings. Little evidence exists for this but it is reasonable to question whether there can there be too much access.

Anecdotal accounts from some of the early walk-in centres suggest that repeat attenders with problems that would be better dealt with in a general practice are a problem,[35] whereas other users may have self-limiting complaints that do not require medical or nursing input. Hutchison[36] has suggested that public education interventions may be a better way to promote self-care than walk-in clinics. However, communicating distinctions about 'appropriate' use of care to patients is difficult, as attested by the numbers of attendances in general practice and walk-in centres for minor self-limiting problems. The choice to attend for a consultation with a health professional, in whatever setting, is a complex one and is not always related to the severity or chronicity of the presenting complaint.

In a similar debate over 'inappropriate' use of A&E departments in the 1980s and 1990s, it became clear that the service itself had to alter in order to meet users' needs – rather than trying to educate users to use primary care in certain circumstances instead of the A&E service.[37] Primary care doctors were therefore sited within A&E departments, and most evidence seems to suggest better use of A&E resources as a result. It remains unclear whether a similar level of cost-effectiveness will eventually be attributed to NHS Direct and walk-in centres, or whether, as some critics argue, the resources devoted to these services would produce greater clinical benefits elsewhere. Moreover, the answer to these questions will depend in part on the value attributed to the convenient and timely access they offer their users.

EFFECTIVENESS AND COST-EFFECTIVENESS

Questions on the effectiveness of recent access innovations depend, of course, on their particular aims. For instance, NHS Direct has been found to be popular with users but the effect on demand management with respect to the Health Service as a whole remains unevaluated. More fundamentally, effectiveness in terms of improved health status is even less clear. This is an important question for all the access policies described above, but one that is methodologically extremely complex to address.

In the final evaluation of NHS Direct, questions were raised about the cost-effectiveness of the service, which remain to be answered.[38] No cost-effectiveness data is yet available on walk-in centres but there are some lessons to be learned from international experience, particularly in Canada,[39,40] where walk–in centres developed from the late 1970s onwards. The centres represent about 3 per cent of total first contact health expenditure and deal mainly with minor ailments. They are cheaper than A&E care but similar in cost to general practice. Overall, there is little evidence for their effectiveness or economic impact. In general, for this raft of policies, it is only if the specific access aims are made clear – absolute or relative – and appropriate evaluation and monitoring put in place, that the answers to this and other (cost-) effectiveness issues will become clear. So far this has not happened.

ACCESS TO SECONDARY CARE

In addition to the primary care policies described above, there are a number of new initiatives aimed at improving access to secondary care. These include 'collaboratives', 'action on' programmes,

elements of the national service frameworks and the work of NPAT. Central to these initiatives – which focus on a single intervention (e.g. cataract), whole specialties (e.g. A&E, orthopaedics) or clusters of diseases (e.g. cancers) – are programmes of organisational redesign. These aim to increase organisational efficiency, reduce unnecessary hospital visits by patients and generally speed up patient throughput between first visit and final treatment. The NHS Plan adds to these initiatives – with a particular focus on improving the timeliness and throughput of patient contacts with acute hospitals.

In this section we consider how two of these initiatives – both prominent in the NHS Plan – might actually affect access: the National Booked Admissions Programme (NBAP) and the introduction of two-week waits for outpatient appointments for those with suspected cancer.

We pay particular attention to the balance these schemes may achieve between absolute and relative access, noting existing research findings that timely entrance into the hospital system is not necessarily followed by equitable and timely access to investigation and treatment. We also discuss the methodological complexity of assessing the impact of these innovations both on different aspects of access and on overall health outcomes. We consider mechanisms for putting some of these initiatives into practice and highlight some of the tensions between improving absolute versus relative access.

BOOKED ADMISSIONS

The NBAP is a large programme of innovation designed to bring booked admissions throughout the NHS by 2005. This was one of the key programmes started by NPAT and now brought under the overall leadership of the Modernisation Board and Agency. The initiatives aim to 'make booking a hospital admission … as easy as booking an airline ticket'.[41]

Guidance has been produced on methods for implementing a booked admissions programme. Several hundred separate projects are now underway. A report on NBAP[42] describes the methods used and some of the problems and issues that have arisen as the programmes have been implemented. Teams work with regional and local managers to identify the services where booked admissions are to be introduced and to train those working on the ground. Milestones set in the 2000/01 Implementation Programme for the NHS Plan were that 'by March 2001 every acute trust should be booking at least two specialities or high volume procedures' and 'by March 2002, 5 million patients would have benefited from the Booked Admissions programme'.[43]

From the early evaluation it is evident that such a programme can substantially reduce the number of stages a patient has to go through before being admitted to hospital as an elective patient (referral–outpatient appointment–waiting list–pre-admission assessment–admission *versus* referral–outpatient appointment with booking for admission–admission).[44]

However, in line with policy guidance, much work on booked admissions has concentrated to date on day-case procedures. A report on booked admissions systems for inpatient care[45] drew the following conclusions:

- elective admissions overall would have to be waiting less than six months and outpatient waiting times would have to reduce to make booking systems viable
- sufficient capacity would be needed to ring-fence elective admissions and allow emergency admissions to be dealt with separately to reduce the chance of cancellations to zero
- operating theatres would have to have extended running times with greater staff flexibility and increased staff cover to enable hospitals to cope with peaks of demand

and, as a more general conclusion arising from the above observations:

- the introduction of a totally booked system would require a major organisational and cultural change programme

This last and most general conclusion demonstrates the importance of taking a system-wide view of organisational developments, such as the introduction of booked admissions in the acute sector. There may be considerable and unanticipated knock-on effects throughout an acute trust when implementing booked admissions. For example, new processes will be required for dealing with emergencies and planning operating theatre schedules, and failure to address these issues could disrupt other services.

Any evaluation of the health impact of booked admissions would have to take into account all the consequences – both intended and unintended – of its introduction. Research is needed to quantify the relative health benefits of ring-fencing elective care compared with systems that more flexibly mix elective and emergency care according to relative demand. However, such research would be methodologically complex; it might be problematic to deal adequately with subtle changes in case mix or in emergency hospitalisation rates, and it is by no means clear that there would be positive health benefits compared to a system that maintained flexibility of response to emergency demand.

In summary, booked admissions undoubtedly increase absolute access to, and convenience of care, and a huge programme is underway to implement them. The NHS is well on target to ensure that by 2005 all elective admissions are booked in advance. However, research to date highlights the potential for important and unpredicted knock-on effects of such a programme across the wider hospital. Furthermore, conclusions about whether the programme actually improves access may depend on which definition of access is adopted for evaluation. Certainly, relative access is likely to be improved by any process that reduces the number of steps required before a person is admitted to hospital. But it remains debatable and as yet unresearched as to whether booked admissions improve a population's overall health.

TWO-WEEK CANCER WAITS

The introduction of two-week cancer waits most obviously aims to improve absolute access to cancer specialists. Some of the key questions here are: whether the initiative will also improve access to the next stages of care after initial diagnosis (i.e. cancer treatment and palliation); how it will affect relative access; and whether it will contribute to improved health outcomes.

The two-week standard is designed to improve timely access into the hospital

system, but does not address the subsequent journey through investigations and treatment after first entry. Patients may be referred promptly and receive prompt surgery, only to find long waiting lists for radiotherapy. Within cancer services, therefore, it may be that the two-week standard diverts efforts away from other service areas where improved access is required.

Also important are concerns about relative access to hospital services. First is the possibility that patients with different health problems will wait longer. Overall, 24 per cent of NHS patients in the last quarter of 2000/01 waited more than 13 weeks for their outpatient appointment.[46] This was a particular problem for trauma and orthopaedics patients, where 42 per cent waited more than 13 weeks.

Second is a concern about inequity in access to subsequent hospital care. If the two-week standard for cancer patients were implemented universally, differences in the use of cancer outpatient services between socio-demographic groups (according to age, gender, ethnicity, class, etc.) might reflect differences in need, patient behaviour or the rates at which GPs consider cancer as a differential diagnosis. However, the Plan does not focus on access to care after entering the cancer outpatient system. Various authors have noted differences in treatment rates according to gender[47] and ethnicity.[48] Research is needed to monitor and describe inequalities in relative access to treatment once patients are within the hospital system, as this could undermine any beneficial effects of the two-week standard for selected subgroups of the population.

How might two-week cancer waits affect health outcomes? Reductions in delay are thought to result in reduced likelihood of morbidity and mortality, though these effects are likely to be small. While there is evidence for this assertion in relation to breast cancer, it has not been found to be true for patients with some other cancers.[49,50] Reductions in delay are also likely to result in reduced anxiety and a reduced likelihood of non-attendance. Two-week waits are therefore likely to benefit people with cancer – even if with only small effects.

For people who do not turn out to have cancer, referral to hospital in accordance with the two-week cancer standard may unnecessarily increase anxiety. This may, however, be offset by a rapid definitive exclusion of a cancer diagnosis. Furthermore, if a GP fails to recognise the risk of cancer, a patient may be seen more slowly. And appointments for people with other serious disorders, requiring urgent attention, may be delayed as a result of the two-week standard. This highlights how changes in one part of an outpatient appointment system can affect other parts of the same service.

Certain performance indicators for the NHS Plan aim to examine the two-week standard by monitoring waiting times for patients with breast cancer. An example is seen in a proposed indicator that compares waiting times for patients with breast cancer who are not referred under the two-week standard with those who are.[51]

In summary, though not yet evaluated, the two-week standard is very likely to improve absolute access for people with cancer. Key questions remain, however, about how the standard operates in practice and its knock-on effects on outpatient systems. The Implementation Programme for the NHS Plan for 2001/02[52] mentions two-week waits for

patients referred urgently with suspected cancers to say only that they should be maintained. But it is worth questioning whether more health benefits might have accrued if the effort put into two-week cancer waits had instead been put into reducing waiting times for outpatient appointments in trauma and orthopaedics or into improving access to subsequent hospital care once patients are actually diagnosed with cancer.

OVERCOMING PROBLEMS: THE CONCEPT OF REDESIGN

Recognising that 'whole systems' approaches are needed to implement these innovations, the concept of 'business process re-engineering' (BPR), 're-engineering' or 'redesign' of health care organisations has started to diffuse from the business sector. Recent reports from the NHS emphasise the need for systematic approaches to improving services, a willingness to challenge established methods of practice and the need for a strong patient focus.[53] In many ways, 'redesign' may offer the best chance of improving all aspects of access to hospital care.

WHAT WILL THE NHS PLAN DELIVER IN RELATION TO ACCESS?

With an extensive infrastructure developed to oversee implementation of the NHS Plan, there are strong expectations for change and 'delivery'. Regional access task forces, NPAT and collaboratives are all involved in supporting the implementation of initiatives to improve access. Early reports from some of these groups show that small gains are accruing,[54,55] but the methodology through which change is achieved – testing change on a small scale using Plan Do Study Act (PDSA) cycles – is inherently incremental and the size of the overall task is enormous. It remains to be seen whether enough progress is made to satisfy public demand for better access.

Furthermore, success needs to be critically evaluated. Progress made in advanced access in primary care has attracted both praise and criticism. Some of the participating GPs have been unable to cope with the additional workload and pressures created by the advanced access programme. The work of the cancer collaboratives has raised questions about whether achieving the two-week standards will result in better clinical outcomes.[56]

Reflecting on the particular focus of this chapter on absolute and relative access, further questions arise about the balance that will be obtained between better absolute access due to increased overall provision of services and changes – for better or worse – in relative access for different socio-cultural groups.

The NHS has been notoriously bad at monitoring relative access.[57] Developing *and using* the information systems required to evaluate changes in relative access that follow from implementation of the NHS Plan is essential. Some such measures are included in the proposed NHS performance indicators,[58] but these will not discriminate fully between the many factors that determine relative access (including ethnicity, class, geographic location, etc.). Furthermore, they do not address the more subtle aspects of inequalities in access that were highlighted above such as differences in access to subsequent investigation and treatment after an initial outpatient consultation.

A sophisticated research programme will be required to evaluate the impact of initiatives to improve access resulting from the NHS Plan. This will have to combine measurement of changed *use* of health services with careful evaluation of the experiences of different groups of patients that enter primary and secondary health care, to examine their subsequent experiences and health outcomes. Such research will be commissioned,[59] but as always the mismatch between research and policy time frames will make it hard for findings to influence implementation of the NHS Plan.

1 Murray M. Modernising the NHS. Patient care: access. *BMJ* 2000; 320: 1594–6.

2 Royal College of Physicians. *Acute medicine: the physician's role – proposals for the future.* London: Royal College of Physicians, 2000.

3 Goddard M, Smith P. *Equity of access to health care.* York: University of York, 1998.

4 Demand management learning set web site. *http://www.rddphru.cam.ac.uk/east/demand/demand.htm* (updated November 2000).

5 Florin D. Improving access to primary care. In: Gillam S, editor. *What has New Labour done for primary care? A balance sheet.* London: King's Fund, 2001.

6 Royal College of General Practitioners. *Access to the NHS. Consultation document 3. Proposals for changes to the delivery of health services in England.* A contribution to the 'Modernisation' review, 2000.

7 Department of Health. *The new NHS. Modern, dependable.* London: Department of Health, 1997.

8 Secretary of State for Health. *The NHS Plan: a plan for investment; a plan for reform.* Cm 4818-I. London: The Stationery Office: 17.

9 Department of Health. *NHS performance indicators: a consultation.*

London: Department of Health, 2001.

10 Although see Rosen R, Florin D, Dixon J. *Access to health care. Taking forward the findings from the scoping exercise.* London: King's Fund, 2001. (Commissioned by the National Co-ordinating Centre for Service Delivery and Organisation, London School of Hygiene and Tropical Medicine.) Available at *http://www.lshtm.ac.uk/php/hsru/sdo/cofccall.htm*

11 Fisher B. Wells Park Health Project. In: Heritage Z, editor. *Community participation in primary care. RCGP Occasional Paper 64.* London: Royal College of General Practitioners, 1994.

12 Gulliford M, Hughes D *et al. Access to health care. Report of a scoping exercise.* London: King's College London, 2001. (Commissioned by the National Co-ordinating Centre for Service Delivery and Organisation, London School of Hygiene and Tropical Medicine.)

13 Beecham L. UK Government proposes Health Action Zones. *BMJ* 1997; 315: 7.

14 NHS Executive. *Health Living Centres.* Leeds: NHS Executive, 1999.

15 Department of Health. *Focusing on delivery.* London: Department of Health, 2001.

16 Murray M, 2000. *Op. cit.*

17 Munro J, Nicholl J, O'Cathain A, Knowles E. *Evaluation of NHS Direct first wave sites. First interim report to the Department of Health.* Sheffield: University of Sheffield, School of Health and Related Research, Medical Care Research Unit, 1998.

18 Munro J, Nicholl J, O'Cathain A, Knowles E. *Evaluation of NHS Direct first wave sites. Second interim report to the Department of Health.* Sheffield: University of Sheffield, School of Health and Related Research, Medical Care Research Unit, 2000.

19 Munro J, Nicholl J, O'Cathain A, Knowles E. *Evaluation of NHS Direct first wave sites. Final report of the phase 1 research.* University of Sheffield, School of Health and Related Research, Medical Care Research Unit, 2001.

20 Airey C, Burster S, Erens B, Lilley S-J, Pickering K, Pitson L. *National surveys of NHS patients. General practice 1998* Leeds: NHS Executive, 1999.

21 Munro J *et al.*, 1998. *Op. cit.*

22 Royal College of General Practitioners, 2000. *Op. cit.*

23 *http://www.doh.gov.uk/nhswalkincentres/questions.htm*

24 Mountford L, Rosen R. *NHS walk-in centres in London: an initial assessment.* London: King's Fund, 2001.

25 *Ibid.*

26 Wootton R. Recent advances: telemedicine. *BMJ* 2001; 323: 557–60.

27 *http://www.npdt.org/advancedaccess/introduction.htm*

28 Hastings A, Rao M. Doctoring deprived areas cannot rely on exceptional people. *BMJ* 2001; 323: 409–10.

29 Lewis R, Gillam S, Jenkins C, editors. *Personal medical services pilots: modernising primary care?* London: King's Fund, 2001.

30 McNulty S, Booler T. Waning GP interest in PMS threatens government target. *Pulse* 2001; August 18.

31 Airey C *et al.*, 1999. *Op. cit.*

32 Drummond N, McConnachie A, O'Donnell C, Moffat K J, Wilson P, Ross S. Social variations in reasons for contacting general practice out-of-hours: implications for daytime service provision? *British Journal of General Practice* 2000; 50: 460–4.

33 Salisbury C. Out-of-hours care: ensuring accessible high quality care for all groups of patients. *British Journal of General Practice* 2000; 50: 443–4.

34 Shipman C, Addington-Hall J, Barclay S, Briggs J, Cox I, Daniels L, Millar D. Providing palliative care in primary care: how satisfied are GPs and district nurses with current out-of-hours arrangements. *British Journal of General Practice* 2000; 50: 477–8.

35 Clews G. One step at a time. *BMJ News Review*. 27 May 2000: 18–20.

36 Hutchison B. The place of walk-in clinics in healthcare systems. Uncertainty about impact demands careful evaluation and policy making. *BMJ* 2000; 321: 909–10.

37 Salisbury C, Dale J, Hallam J, editors. *24-hour primary care*. Oxford: Radcliffe Medical Press, 1999.

38 Munro J et al., 2001. *Op. cit.*

39 Hutchison B, 2000. *Op. cit.*

40 Jones M. Lessons from Canada. *BMJ* 2000; 321: 928–31.

41 Meredith P, Ham C et al. *Modernising the NHS: booking patients for hospital care: first interim report from the evaluation of the National Booked Admissions Programme*. Birmingham: University of Birmingham, School of Public Policy, Health Services Management Centre, 1999.

42 *Ibid.*

43 Department of Health. *Implementation programme for the NHS Plan 3. Priorities guidance: provisional milestones and outcomes for 2001/2002*. London: Department of Health, 2000.

44 Meredith P, Ham C et al., 1999. *Op. cit.*

45 Bensley D, Halsall J, McIlwain C, Scott L. *Total booking systems for elective admission*. Department of Health Internal Report. Quoted in Meredith P, Ham C, Kipping R.

46 NHS Executive. *A step-by-step guide to improving out-patient services. Variations in outpatients performance project report II*. London: Department of Health, 2000.

47 Raine R. *Does gender bias exist in the use of specialist health care?* PhD thesis: London School of Hygiene and Tropical Medicine, Department of Public Health & Policy. London: University of London, 2000.

48 Goddard M, Smith P, 1998. *Op. cit.*

49 Richards M, Westcombe A, Love S, Littlejohns P, Ramirez A. Influence of delay on survival in patients with breast cancer: a systematic review. *Lancet* 1999; 353 (9159): 1119–26.

50 Jones R, Rubin G et al. Is the two week rule for cancer referrals working? *BMJ* 2001; 322: 1555–6.

51 Department of Health, 2000, *Op. cit.*

52 Department of Health, 2000, *Op. cit.*

53 See, for example, Locock L. *Maps and journeys: the process of redesign in the NHS*. Birmingham: University of Birmingham, Health Services Management Centre, 2001.

54 Oldham J. *Advance access in primary care*. Manchester: Primary Care Development Team, 2001.

55 National Patients Access Team. *Business plan 2000/2001*. Leicester: NHS Executive, 2000.

56 Rosen R et al., 2001. *Op. cit.*

57 Rosen R et al., 2001. *Op. cit.*

58 Department of Health, 2001. *Op. cit.*

59 Rosen R et al., 2001. *Op. cit*

Delivering the NHS Plan: a case of 'constrained innovation'

Jacky Eyres and Steve Dewar

INTRODUCTION

A plan is one thing, delivery quite another. The question of how best to achieve planned change across a complex organisation such as the NHS is one that successive political leaders have had to address. For some time, civil servants in the Department of Health have compared the management tools available for effecting change to 'rubber levers which when pushed bend in the middle but effect little change on the ground'.[1] But this time the stakes are high. For politicians, a contemporary answer to the problem holds the key to electoral survival. For the NHS, Tony Blair believes it is 'reform or bust'.[2] Public and patient expectations are high and disappointment would be palpable.

How does one create the climate that encourages (or even ensures) delivery of the NHS Plan?[3] The current UK approach is characterised by two dominant groupings of words, ideas and rhetoric. The first emphasises the use of a centralised command and control approach to reform. As the Prime Minister acknowledged, 'in our first term there was heavy intervention from the centre'.[4] This is evident in new national standards, national evaluation of new treatments, new structures for national inspection and regulation – and new frameworks of accountability. It is characterised by a concern to extend or tighten the *grip* over managers, services or outcomes.

The second set of ideas, words and rhetoric emphasises changes to 'devolve power and responsibility to frontline organisations', 'empowering' frontline staff, making them 'architects of public service reform', putting them in the 'driving seat of change' – in short, a freeing up of managerial and professional creativity and *space*. As Alan Milburn has put it, 'the time has now come to free the NHS frontline'.[5,6]

There may be tension between these two approaches. Each, on its own, postulates a different underlying model of delivery. One stresses the need to enforce accountability for delivering pre-determined outcomes and targets – while not necessarily acknowledging the complexity and innovation that characterises successful policy implementation. The other implies that the desired change will flow from freeing up that very potential for individual and organisational innovation while playing down the directed and determined nature of national reform.

The potential for this tension to become counterproductive is acknowledged by many. Even the Secretary of State noted that, while national standards are necessary, some feel that centralisation has crowded out innovation and left staff feeling 'disempowered' by the process. Cabinet Office papers went further, recognising that 'excessively directive methods of government that appear to treat front-line deliverers as unable to think for themselves, untrustworthy or incompetent, undermine the very motivation and adaptability on which real-world success depends'.[7] Government acknowledges that 'getting the balance right is never easy'.[8]

But the apparent contradictory nature of the two approaches may not be a problem. Indeed, many leaders advocate what are sometimes called 'loose–tight' frameworks combining clear objectives with local freedom to adopt local solutions. In the round, health policy initiatives can be seen as attempting to take this approach – combining elements of grip (centralisation, command and control, and tight performance management) with space (empowerment and individual and local responsibility). 'Freeing the frontline' is presented within a framework of strong national objectives and accountability.

The new emphasis on freedom is not an abandonment of previous centralisation and control. As Rudolf Klein commented when Alan Milburn announced

government intentions to shift the balance of power to frontline organisations, 'this is an attempt to inject freedom in a way that allows innovation in the knowledge that liberty is not a licence for poor standards or inadequate performance'.[9] Indeed, a recent Commission for Health Improvement (CHI) report warned of the dangers of 'semi-autonomous fiefdoms' in hospitals.[10] And the Kennedy inquiry into children's heart surgery at the Bristol Royal Infirmary criticised the high level of unaccountable devolution in that Trust.[11] These are examples of the potential negative consequences of freedoms that might give space for innovation but end up hiding poor practice.

To describe New Labour's approach to combining space and grip, we offer the phrase 'constrained innovation'. It suggests the potential contradiction and paradox inherent in this particular 'third way' and encapsulates some of the tensions inherent in combining the twin ideas of greater 'grip' over the pace and direction of change, and more 'space' for the necessary innovation required to get there. The question is, will this prove to be a synergistic solution to the problem of delivery, or will this characteristic New Labour stance collapse under contradictory rhetoric?

MODERNISATION AND 'CONSTRAINED INNOVATION'

The NHS Plan is clear about its desire to change the culture of the NHS. This process of change is often labelled as 'modernisation'. This attempt to change culture is highly directed – the characteristics of the new culture are repeatedly listed (patient centred, accessible, quality assured, and so on) and a proliferation of national initiatives are working to help stimulate and direct change, as well as to assess achievements against national criteria. Commentators note that, in building a strong culture, an organisation often constrains the options available to people in a conscious attempt to direct change and reduce the incidence of random response.[12]

This can leave less room for individuals to manoeuvre or to depart from common practice – even innovation itself can become constrained and directed, determined more by organisational rules than individual creativity. What can be done is delimited by the cultural milieu – 'the way we do things round here'. Entrepreneurial (or risk-taking) behaviour itself becomes a risky business, as deviation from organisational norms can bring severe sanction. Perversely, there is a danger that the approach being taken to establish an NHS culture that might foster innovation ends up constraining it.

'Constrained innovation' describes a restrained and regulated approach to change. It implies that the need for innovation is put within the straitjacket of a tight timetable and robust framework of performance management, driven by the aims and objectives of a strong culture change project. The demands of central planning leave NHS managers and organisations with limited freedom to innovate – the component parts of innovation come flat-packed in the shape of national service frameworks (NSFs) and the like. Within 'constrained innovation' there is still an expectation of new ideas, processes and services. The difference is in the detailed specification of the outcome that precedes the act of innovation.

The language of modernisation embraces newness, creativity, innovation and progress – these are all deemed positives. However, the more disconcerting notion of unpredictable change – ideas of chance, of indeterminacy, of unforeseeability – that lurks within the very concept of change or newness means that it has to be carefully managed and bounded in case it runs out of control. This control is provided through the monitoring and standard setting roles of bodies such as CHI and the National Institute of Clinical Excellence (NICE) – two key agencies of modernisation.

However, with too strong a hand on the tiller there is a risk that 'constrained innovation' fails to tap into a more 'genuine innovation' that is creative, passionate, personal and owned. This type of innovation may not be responsive to directive and timetable: rather it stems from wellsprings within an organisation, both collective and individual. It frequently draws on local and tacit knowledge – concepts that are receiving increasing attention in terms of organisational learning.[13]

THE NHS PLAN AND THE TWIN IDEAS OF 'GRIP' AND 'SPACE'

The rhetoric of the NHS Plan and subsequent policy such as 'Shifting the Balance' implies a new deal for NHS managers (as well as frontline professional staff with managerial responsibilities). An outline of this type of deal is provided by Christopher Hood, a leading writer on regulation and public management, who claims that such a new bargain between the heads of public service organisations and politicians is at the heart of many contemporary ambitions to reform public services.[14] Hood states that the deal exchanges extra responsibility for executives with a commitment from politicians to abjure hands-on control – 'politicians give up the right to roam at will within public servants' "free managerial space"'. He stresses that:

> In these conditions there is far more emphasis on controlling public servants according to output and outcome rather than only on input and process, and hence more scope for 'results-based' approaches to public management.[14]

Hood goes on to outline the consequences in terms of a set of regulatory entailments with a strong but arm's-length regulatory process. The combination of national standards (through the Plan, the work of NICE and the NSFs) with strong regulatory bodies (such as CHI) certainly accords with this description of a new type of public service bargain. The Bristol Inquiry report also talks about the need for CHI to have sufficient independence, authority and available sanctions (or regulatory grip) to fulfil its role. Recent government policy focuses on the attempt to create more managerial space. Taken together, these seem to present a coherent framework to direct the delivery of change through a new managerial bargain combining regulatory grip, national objectives and increased managerial autonomy.

However, this coherence may be illusory. The approach outlined by Hood suggests that an increase in regulatory grip might be accompanied by a corresponding loosening of the central chain of organisational command, the relationships between the two different types of burden (regulatory and 'hands-on' direction) being in inverse proportion – mirror images of each other. Indeed, the commitment in the NHS Plan to reduce the number of government circulars going to the NHS, from one a day, to one a week, signalled a willingness to accept this part of the bargain. But, instead, there is evidence of an even greater use of central mechanisms of control in an understandable attempt to drive delivery forward over a short term, politically determined timetable.[15]

Given the high political stakes, one can understand the temptation to impose more and more ways to try and ensure the delivery of change. Hood calls this a 'double whammy' pattern of regulation, where public managers are subject to more process rules *and* more regulation of other types. However, if not in balance, the co-existence of these two different frameworks of direction and accountability can confuse the question of who is responsible for change. The new public service bargain is vulnerable to those who want to pass the buck. Politicians can attempt to control and direct, while trying to shift the blame for the consequences of that influence to managers: managers can politicise any evaluation of their performance, pointing to the constrained circumstances that make the delivery of cumulative targets impossible.

Some regulatory commentators suggest that a type of variable regulation might help ensure delivery without squashing initiative and innovation. In health care, such ideas lie behind the development of 'earned autonomy'. Hood describes such an approach as one in which regulators leave regulatees to write their own rules except when the latter are seen by the former as delinquent or failing'. However, if the autonomy that can be earned is to be substantial then this too will require a culture that can tolerate substantial discretion and variation between organisations. The danger here is that the impact of labelling trusts 'good' or 'poor' on the basis of national targets will become the dominant part of the earned autonomy system. This would reinforce the sense of regulatory grip over the delivery of a centrally driven agenda and detract from the very autonomy that might be earned. Achieving the right balance in any system of 'constrained innovation' is difficult. Indeed, in this case public statements of success or failure may make many managers feel less inclined to take the risks that innovation requires.

'CONSTRAINED INNOVATION': CONSEQUENCES AND IMPLICATIONS

There are three potential untoward consequences of 'constrained innovation'. First, it carries the danger of de-incentivising managers. Instead of producing commitment and enthusiasm for change, a strong centralised drive for delivery with sanctions for non-achievement can engender a superficial compliance without real engagement and innovation. Some commentators suggest that such situations discourage a deep identification with corporate goals and values, and instead lead to the development of a selective, calculative compliance.[16]

Second, there is the problem of creating enough space to allow for genuine innovation. If the management agenda is taken up with implementing top-down change and responding to the 'double whammy' of profuse 'orders of the day' and strong regulatory requirements, then what room is left for the sort of innovation that comes from activities such as reflection, discussion and networking? It has been suggested that organisations with a successful record of innovation have a degree of 'slack' –

uncommitted resources of people, finance, material and motivation.[17] When there is slack, the psychological risk of new ventures is reduced – the possible loss of uncommitted resources is less painful than the loss of resources that are already earmarked for specific use. This is highly relevant to the NHS, which has little slack in any of its resources.

Third, to what extent does 'constrained innovation' rest on a misunderstanding of the concept of change? The current agenda for change relies on an assumption that innovation diffuses through an organisational network. An idea may be poured into the top of the system and trickle its way through, permeating all of the organisational nooks and crannies. An alternative to this is the translation model of innovation, which suggests that an idea or practice makes its way between the nodes of a network, sometimes passing easily between them, at other times encountering resistance.[18] Crucially, at each twist and turn the innovation becomes in some way altered as the various elements of the network translate and hence transform it. On this view it is only to be expected that an innovation will undergo en route change that is outside the control of the centre that issued it – it is subject to the local and the contingent. No matter how much the centre seeks to maintain control of the innovation, it will find its ultimate expression in the hands of its end-users, or implementers.

NEW LABOUR: THE NEED FOR EXPERIMENT AND LEARNING

Tony Blair's mantra that 'what counts is what works' implies considerable scope for innovation – but only to achieve the goal of a 'working' service that is often defined in terms of national standards. Such 'constrained innovation' is typical of New Labour's approach. On the positive side it shows concern with change and improvement – it is active and well intended. It is linked to a clear political commitment – NHS change is at the top of the Government's agenda and there is (for now) funding to accompany the call for change. However, working out how to make 'constrained innovation' work means learning how to achieve an effective balance between central grip and managerial space.

The New Labour approach includes many initiatives that combine grip and space in different proportions. Primary care groups (PCGs) and primary care trusts (PCTs) are classic hybrids of this type – representing a balance between power and space for primary care communities to influence new service development while pulling quite isolated and disparate practitioners into stronger systems of accountability. Policy interest in networks and partnerships also fit this picture – they are approaches that seek to enlarge the local playing field for change, creating new space within which clinicians and managers can innovate. Yet they also strive towards national standards and create new structures within which managers and clinicians can be held to account.

These new approaches to change show innovation at the heart of government. However, one characteristic of innovation is that not every approach will be successful. The challenge is to learn from success as well as allowing and learning from failure. To facilitate this process it may be helpful to give some bodies (such as individual PCGs or PCTs) an exception from some of the norms of national grip so that they can experiment and take risks. This would improve our chances of learning how to mix and match the concepts of grip and space in a way that can really encourage innovation and delivery within a national service.

The Government, public and Health Service know that having a plan is one thing and delivery is quite another. 'Constrained innovation' describes the policy path of choice. It may or may not prove to be an effective framework for the necessary scale of national change. Learning from experiment and experience will be crucial. But the stakes are high; if delivery is delayed the consequent disillusion will spell electoral danger for the Government, a turbulent future for the NHS, and dashed expectations for public and patient alike.

1   Rhodes A W. *The Economic and Social Research Council's Whitehall Programme: the governance narrative*. Newcastle: University of Newcastle, 2001.
2   Prime Minister. *Public service reform*. Speech at the Royal Free Hospital, 16 July 2001.
3   Secretary of State. *The NHS Plan: a plan for investment; a plan for reform*. Cm 4818-I. London: Stationery Office, 2000.
4   *Ibid*.
5   Department of Health. *Shifting the balance of power within the NHS: securing delivery*. Leeds: Department of Health, 2001.
6   Milburn A. *Shifting the balance of power in the NHS*. Speech to mark the launch of the Modernisation Agency, 25 April 2001.
7   Cabinet Office, Performance and Innovation Unit. *Better policy delivery and design: a discussion paper*. London: 2001.
8   Department of Health, 2001. *Op. cit.*
9   Klein R. Milburn's vision of a new NHS: adopting the missionary position. *BMJ* 2001; 322: 1078–9.
10 Commission for Health Improvement.

Investigation into issues arising from the case of Loughborough GP Peter Green. London: Stationery Office, 2001.

11 Learning from Bristol: the report of the public inquiry into children's heart surgery at the Bristol Royal Infirmary 1984–1995. Cmnd 5207. London: Stationery Office, 2001.

12 Mangham I, Pye A. *The doing of managing.* Oxford: Blackwell Business, 1991.

13 Wenger E C, Snyder W M. Communities of practice: the organizational frontier. *Harvard Business Review* 2001; Jan–Feb: 139–45.

14 Hood C. *The art of the state: culture, rhetoric, and public management.* Oxford: Oxford University Press, 1998.

15 Department of Health. *The NHS Plan implementation programme.* Leeds: Department of Health, 2001.

16 Willmott H. Strength is ignorance; slavery is freedom: managing culture in modern organisations. *Journal of Management Studies* 1993; 30 (4): 515–52.

17 Mueller R K. *The innovation ethic.* New York: American Management Association Inc., 1971.

18 Latour B. Technology is society made durable. In: Law J, editor. *A sociology of monsters: essays on power, technology and domination.* London: Routledge, 1991.

Capacity and service delivery

Pippa Gough

Staff are integral to the success of the Government's modernisation plans. To increase capacity and quality of care there have to be sufficient numbers of appropriately qualified Health Service staff to deliver. Sadly, there are not, particularly within nursing and medicine – a fact that various professional bodies and trade unions have been keen to point out.

The three papers in this section explore the issue of capacity and service delivery from different angles. The first, by Belinda Finlayson, gives an overview of where some of the problems lie and how the Government has responded through a variety of policy initiatives aimed at boosting recruitment and retention. While the Government is satisfied that it will hit most of its staffing targets set out in the NHS Plan,[1] Finlayson argues that these targets fall short of the mark and the demand–supply gap continues to widen. The policy initiatives, although laudable, are not cutting the mustard.

The second paper, by Sandra Meadows and George Blair, focuses on the loss of experience through the leaching away of older staff from our health services – staff who, she argues, are valuable and much needed but who are generally disillusioned, work injured and worn out, and are seeking refuge in early retirement in increasing numbers. Her paper sets out some possible solutions worthy of further examination.

The final paper, by Professor Sir Cyril Chantler, takes a different tack, and concentrates less on the quantity of staff but focuses instead on how existing staff can be used in different ways to boost capacity and provide more appropriate care. This is care suited to the needs of a population that is ageing and requires not so much acute, high-tech intervention but rather rehabilitation, respite and intermediate care. This approach requires a wholesale rethink about the way in which the health workforce is reconfigured and rigid professional boundaries softened and merged. Within intermediate care the dominant therapy is not necessarily medicine – an approach that holds so much sway in our current system – but lies instead with that provided by nurses, therapists and others. Sadly, these are the staff who, within the current way of thinking, have very little say over how patients and users are admitted to, cared for in and discharged from our health system. Because of the Government's preoccupation with numbers, it is this thinking that appears to have failed to permeate the modernising zeal.

The problem is that the health care workforce needs a total rethink if capacity and service delivery is going to match the aspirations set out in the Plan. The message constantly given out by the Government is the need for more patient-centred care, less professional dominance, more teamwork, and less rigid professional hierarchies. In effect, we are talking about a shift in the very models of professionalism upon which our health services are founded. This will not be achieved through the numbers game alone: it requires a more radical and thoughtful approach to changing professional identity and professional culture – changes that strike at the heart of traditional systems of regulation, education, accreditation and pay and reward. We hear the Government talk about this: we do not yet see it reflected fully in its policies. The basic questions about capacity are this: are the professions in their current form (a social construct of the eighteenth century) sustainable in the twenty-first century, and are they suited to the service delivery that is required? The answer has to be: not without significant change. Within a sophisticated, informed, consumerist society, the current professional approach – based on hierarchy, elitism, mastery and paternalism – is approaching clinical, social and ethical bankruptcy. The

numbers game, though important, is not the only key to modernisation. We will need to define the roles of each professional group, what can and cannot be shared, and the education and training required throughout a professional career.

This change, however, is a difficult call for the Government and the Royal Colleges. It is understandable that the politicians hold the focus tightly on quantitative targets and number crunching statistics whenever the workforce issue is raised. After all, hitting targets (however erroneous they may be) wins more political plaudits and votes, and is a whole lot less painful than unpicking the traditions and vested interests of the medical and other health professions – even if this is in the name of improved quality of care and increased responsiveness. The issue of capacity has not yet been addressed. This following section starts the debate on the road to developing a more far-reaching critique.

1   Secretary of State for Health. *The NHS Plan: a plan for investment; a plan for reform.* Cm 4818-I. London: Stationery Office, 1997.

The recruitment and retention challenge

Belinda Finlayson

Staff are the lifeblood of the NHS. They will underpin the success (or failure) of the Government's plans to modernise the NHS. But they are in a bad way; key professions are struggling to

attract new recruits and facing an even tougher battle to retain existing staff. Beyond the NHS, the public sector as a whole is becoming less appealing as a place to work.[1] The Government has responded with a variety of initiatives from boosting pay to improving the working lives of staff.

This paper will outline the recruitment and retention problems across three staff groups – nurses and midwives, doctors and therapists. It will then outline the policy response to these problems and assess whether the efforts are adequate.

RECRUITMENT AND RETENTION

NURSES AND MIDWIVES

The Labour Government which came to power in 1997 inherited a sick patient from its Conservative predecessor. Nursing and midwifery training numbers were severely cut in the early to mid-1990s and began to recover only towards the end of that decade. This had an impact on both the number of nurses and midwives qualifying and joining the nursing and midwifery register, and on the volume of nurses and midwives able to be employed in the NHS.

The NHS in England employs 256,280 WTE registered nurses, registered midwives and health visitors, and a further 10,710 WTE registered nurses working in general practice (though more are directly employed by GPs). There were 634,529 nurses and midwives registered with the nursing and midwifery professional body, the UK Central Council for Nursing, Midwifery and Health Visiting (UKCC), at the end of March 2000.[2]

The NHS also employs 23,140 WTE health care assistants, who may have trained to the level of National Vocational Qualifications (NVQ) but, although considered part of the wider nursing workforce, are not registered with the UKCC.[3]

Figure 1 shows changes in the number of UKCC registrants since 1990.

Figure 1: UKCC total registrants, 1990–2001

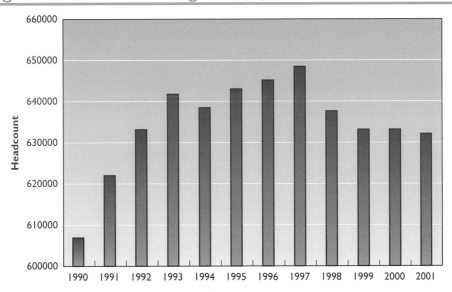

Source: UKCC. Annual statistics. Volume 1. 2000; UKCC. Big increase in new UK-trained nurses on national register. Press release, 3 May 2001.

The overall number of registrants is shown to have increased by almost 30,000 between 1990 and 2001, peaking in 1997. However, this obscures two worrying trends. First, the number of *entrants* to the register declined by around a third (6000) between 1990/1 and 1998/9. Second, the number of *leavers* has exceeded the number of *entrants* to the register for the past decade. For example, in 1997/8, 16,392 nurses and midwives joined the register while 27,173 left.[4] There are several possible explanations for this trend:

- it reflects reductions in the number of pre-registration training numbers in the early to mid-1990s
- increasing numbers of nurses are retiring
- changes in post-registration education and practice (PREP) requirements
- overseas nurses and midwives forgoing their membership.

In the future, two further trends are likely to impact on the register. First, the nursing and midwifery workforce is ageing, which means the number of nurses retiring is forecast to double from 5500 a year at present to more than 10,000 a year by 2005.[5] Second, the number of overseas-trained nurses joining the register is likely to outstrip the number of UK-trained nurses, partly as a result of government recruitment campaigns to boost nursing numbers (discussed later).

Two ways to measure staff retention are:

- through the number of staff vacancies (which are typically measured as a snapshot on a particular day of the year)
- staff turnover (the number of staff who have left a post in a particular trust over one year).

The latest NHS Vacancy Survey suggests there were around 9000 nurse vacancies at the end of March 2001, 1000 less than the year before.[6] However, the NHS Vacancy Survey includes only those vacant posts that NHS trusts have been actively trying to fill for three months or more. The Royal College of Nursing (RCN) has also calculated vacancy rates. By counting an established post as vacant the moment it becomes unfilled and also including posts that have been frozen, the RCN estimates the real vacancy rate is nearer 22,000 WTE.[7]

The former Education and Training Consortia, which planned and commissioned non-medical training places, compiled vacancy and turnover rates for their areas. But there is a dearth of centralised national information on staff turnover rates in the NHS. This makes national workforce planning extremely difficult. There is a possibility that the new Workforce Development Confederations, which have a wider remit than the Consortia they succeeded, could help solve this problem.

DOCTORS

The medical profession is also facing severe shortages, though historically ministers have been less willing to concede this than they have been for nurses. More than 190,000 doctors were registered with the General Medical Council (GMC) in 2000. On average, 9200 join the register each year. Of these, 42 per cent are trained in the UK, 18 per cent in the European Economic Area (EEA) and 40 per cent from elsewhere overseas.[8] Figure 2 shows changes in the number of GMC registrants from 1990.

This figure shows the overall number of registrants increased between 1990 and 2000. However, this masks an interesting

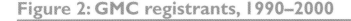

Figure 2: GMC registrants, 1990–2000

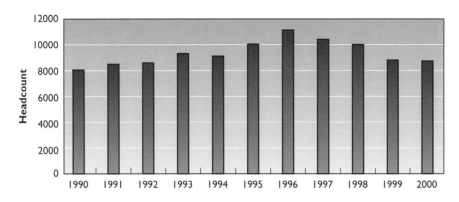

Source: GMC. Personal communication.

trend. While the number of doctors joining the register from training in the UK continued to increase steadily over this period, the number of doctors joining the register who qualified in the EEA and non-EEA countries increased until 1996 but subsequently tapered off. For example, in 1996, 2435 doctors from the EEA and 4715 from non-EEA countries registered to practise in the UK. By 2000, those numbers had declined to 1380 EEA-trained doctors and 2866 non-EEA-trained doctors – a trend that may negatively impact on government plans to recruit overseas' doctors to plug the gaps in the NHS.

The NHS in England employed 57,940 WTE hospital doctors (consultants and doctors in training)[9] and 30,252 (headcount) general practitioners as at September 2000.[10] Results from the latest NHS Vacancy Survey reveal there were 670 consultant vacancies in England in March 2001.[11]

A survey on general practitioner recruitment, retention and vacancy rates revealed there were 1214 GP vacancies in England and Wales at the end of March 2000.[12] This figure looks set to increase as significant numbers of Asian doctors recruited to plug gaps in the 1970s approach retirement. In some health authorities, this could mean a loss of one in four GPs.[13] The number of doctors qualifying as GPs hit an all-time low in 1998. The Joint Committee on Postgraduate Training for General Practice issued only 1663 certificates of qualification that year, compared to 2562 in 1981.[14] By 2000, the number of certificates issued had barely increased to 1689.

Academic medicine is also struggling to attract and retain staff, with 79 vacant chair posts, 145 vacancies for senior lecturers and 177 vacancies for lecturers.[15]

Upstream, the number of applications to medical schools has been falling steadily over the last five years. In 1996, the University and Colleges Admissions Service (UCAS) received 12,025 applications to study medicine. By 1998, that number had dropped to 11,807 applications, and by 2000 it had dropped further to 10,226.[16]

ALLIED HEALTH PROFESSIONALS

The NHS in England employs 40,530 WTE allied health professionals. Of these, the biggest professional groups are physiotherapists at 12,510 WTE, occupational therapists at 11,190 WTE and diagnostic radiographers at 9170 WTE.[17] As at July 2001, there were 133,377 state registered allied health professionals registered with the Council for the Professions Supplementary to Medicine (CPSM) (due to become the new Health Professions Council). Of those, 31,745 are physiotherapists, 22,352 are occupational therapists and 20,341 are diagnostic and therapeutic radiographers.

Figure 3 shows changes in the numbers of allied health professionals registered with CPSM since 1988.

This table shows a steady increase in the numbers of allied health professionals registered with the CPSM from 1988 to 2000. The reason for the sharp increase in registrants between 2000 and 2001 may be that, during this period, three new professional groups were incorporated

into the register: speech and language therapists; clinical scientists; and paramedics.

The NHS Vacancy Survey in 2001 revealed 1820 vacancies among the allied health professional workforce working for the NHS in England, 300 more vacancies than at the same time in the previous year.

THE NHS PLAN

The NHS Plan contained a number of initiatives to modernise NHS staffing, including proposals to boost staffing numbers, improve the working lives of staff and modernise pay, as well as initiatives specific to different staff groups. Each of these is discussed briefly below. Though all laudable, the major challenge for the Government may be to move beyond propping up the existing workforce towards thinking more radically about how the future workforce could be configured differently in order to address the growing gap between demand and supply.

Figure 3: CPSM total registrants, 1988–2001

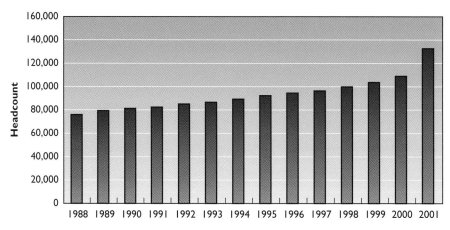

Source: CPSM. Personal communication.

BOOSTING STAFFING NUMBERS

One of the most welcome features of the NHS Plan was the Government's acknowledgement that key professions were suffering recruitment and retention problems – recognition that had long been sought by now-weary professional lobby groups. But it was also a politically astute move by a government that knew the successful implementation of its modernisation agenda would depend on sufficient numbers of (motivated) staff.

The headline figures in the NHS Plan for boosting staffing levels by 2004 at first appeared encouraging – increases of 20,000 nurses, 7500 consultants, 2000 GPs and 6500 therapists. But closer analysis of each of these promises revealed several catches. First, the numbers of nurses are headcount figures, not WTE, which lowers the potential contribution to the NHS. Second, 4500 of the promised extra consultants[18] and 1100 of the 2000 extra GPs[19] were already due to come online. Third, it was clear not all of these places could be met through UK graduates; significant numbers of staff would have to be recruited from overseas to plug the gaps till more UK-trained graduates came online, a point openly conceded by the Government.

Upstream, the Government also promised to increase training places for most staff groups. By 2004, training places for therapists and 'other key professional staff' would increase by 4450 a year. Over the same period, nurse training places would increase by 5500 a year, specialist registrar posts would increase by 1000 places, and general practice training posts by 450. But even these increases may not be enough to deliver the numbers of staff needed over the dictated time period. For example, the RCN estimates there are 22,000 WTE nurse vacancies. They suggest that if retirement and other losses remain at current levels, the NHS will actually need to recruit more than 110,000 nurses by 2004 and less than half of these will come through the education system. The remainder will need to be made up in other ways: for example, encouraging nurses who have left to return and/or recruiting from overseas.[20]

IMPROVING WORKING LIVES

Boosting staffing numbers is only part of the solution; another part lies in retaining existing staff. Realising this, the Government committed itself to a comprehensive range of policies designed to improve the working lives of staff. Many of these initiatives were outlined first in the White Paper *Improving Working Lives*[21] and reiterated in the NHS Plan.

Under the *Improving Working Lives Standard*,[22] which must be met by 2003, NHS employers must prove they are committed to staff training and development; are tackling discrimination and harassment; are acting on the Government's zero-tolerance policy on violence against staff; have a workforce that is representative of the local community; and offer flexible and family-friendly working opportunities.

However, evidence suggests many of these initiatives are taking a long time to translate into tangible services for staff on the ground. Furthermore, a 'worrying' proportion of staff are unaware of the opportunities available to them.[23] And some of the initiatives, such as the target for 100 trusts to have on-site nurseries by 2004, are modest.

INCREASING PAY

Another key plank in the Government's attempts to retain staff has been to address poor levels of pay among public sector workers. Pay is one of the key factors that influence a nurse's decision to leave the NHS,[24] and may also influence the behaviour of other health professionals in a similar way.

Under the Labour Government, nurses have received year-on-year pay increases. In the latest pay round, which took effect from 1 April 2001, nurses were awarded a basic pay increase of 3.7 per cent. Senior nurses, on whom the Government was dependent to implement key aspects of the Plan, were awarded a rise of 5 per cent.[25] At the same time, doctors were awarded a 3.9 per cent rise, while the allied health professions received a 3.7 per cent basic increase. However, the pay of nurses and allied health professionals still lags behind that of other public sector workers. For example, a nurse starts work on £15,445 and a physiotherapist on £15,920. An untrained police officer starts work on £17,133 and a qualified teacher on £16,038 or £17,001 (depending on their level of attainment).[26]

A more recent commitment to invest in pay came in the form of golden 'hellos' and 'goodbyes' for GPs and nurses. Newly qualified GPs would receive a 'golden hello' of £5000, with an extra £5000 if they began work in a deprived area. GPs who waited until they were 65 to retire would receive a £10,000 'golden goodbye'. In addition, nurses, midwives and therapists who took a return to practice course would be entitled to £1000.[27] But the awards were controversial and were described variously by some as something that would make a real difference, for example

to nurses wanting to return to the profession,[28] and by others as a 'golden handcuff'.[29]

NURSES, MIDWIVES AND THERAPISTS

Nurses who have left the NHS often cite limitations to the development of their clinical role as a major source of frustration.[30] Recognising this, a key proposal within the NHS Plan centres on 'breaking down barriers between staff' and enabling different professions to take on new roles. Following the NHS Plan's commitment to encourage new ways of working, the Changing Workforce Programme was set up to pilot different options for doing so.

Another frustration for nurses and therapists has been the historical lack of senior clinical posts – senior posts have tended to be concentrated in management positions.[31] Both the NHS Plan and the earlier *Making a Difference* outlined the Government's commitment to addressing this historical imbalance. *Making a Difference* set out the Government's plans for a modern career framework for nurses, including the creation of 500 consultant posts for nurses, midwives and health visitors. The number of these posts is set to double by 2004, but even this is modest. The Plan also included proposals to 'bring back matron', but it is not yet clear how many such posts will be created.

DOCTORS

While the NHS Plan encouraged career development for nurses and therapists through an expansion of their roles, it simultaneously outlined plans that could potentially curtail the career development of consultants through 'inviting' them to accept a seven-year ban on private practice following graduation or face an expansion of the much reviled sub-consultant grade. Even if this was chiefly added as a bargaining chip, it was an unwise move by a Government that had already recognised its dependence on motivated NHS staff to implement its modernisation agenda.

GPs fared slightly better under the NHS Plan than their consultant colleagues. They received a commitment to upgrade 3000 premises by 2000, earmarked (but unspecified) funds to support continuing professional development, and an entitlement to NHS occupational health services – something they had long campaigned for. Opportunities for GPs to work as salaried doctors rather than independent contractors would be expanded (a move welcomed by some but not by others) and their 'Red Book' GP contract would be revised.

Single-handed GP practices were put under the spotlight (possibly because there had recently been a number of high-profile cases against errant single-handed GPs). In future, they would be subject to new contractual quality standards.

CONCLUSION

The NHS, as well as other parts of the public sector, is experiencing increasing difficulties in recruiting and retaining staff in key professions such as nursing, medicine and the allied health professions. The policy response to these problems has been comprehensive, but the initiatives are taking a long time to translate into tangible services for staff on the ground. Furthermore, the mix of a carrot-and-stick approach has not been well received and may threaten the success of the modernisation agenda. It is unlikely that the Government's

impressive and ambitious targets will be met within the appointed political timeframe.

1 Finlayson B, Dixon J, Meadows S, Blair G. In short supply: the extent of the NHS nursing shortage. Submitted for publication, September 2001.
2 UKCC. Annual statistics. Volume 1. London: UKCC, 2000.
3 Ibid.
4 Ibid.
5 Meadows S, Levenson R, Baeza J. The last straw: explaining the NHS nursing shortage. London: King's Fund, 2000.
6 Department of Health. Statistical bulletin: NHS hospital and community health services non-medical staff in England: 1999–2000. 2001/03. London: Department of Health, 2001.
7 Royal College of Nursing. Making up the difference: a review of the UK nursing labour market in 2000. London: RCN, 2000.
8 General Medical Council. Changing times, changing culture: a review of the work of the GMC since 1995. London: GMC, 2000.
9 Department of Health. Statistical bulletin. 2001/02. London: Department of Health, 2001.
10 Department of Health. Statistical bulletin. 2001/04. London: Department of Health, 2001.
11 Department of Health. Vacancies survey, March 2001. London: Department of Health, 2000.
12 Department of Health. General practitioner recruitment, retention and vacancy survey 2000 for England and Wales. London: Department of Health, 2000.
13 Taylor D, Esmail A. Retrospective analysis of census data on general practitioners who qualified in South Asia: who will replace them as they retire? BMJ 1999; 318: 306–10.
14 Finlayson B. Qualifying GPs hit all-time low. Doctor 1999; 24 June.
15 Robinson F. Wanted! 79 professors, 145

senior lecturers, 177 lecturers. *Hospital Doctor* 2001; 3 August.

16 See *www.ucas.co.uk*

17 Department of Health. *Statistical bulletin: NHS hospital and community health services … Ibid.*

18 Wilson C. Extra posts set to push consultant expansion. *Hospital Doctor* 2000; 3 August.

19 Royal College of General Practitioners. *Position statement on the general practitioner workforce: one of a series of documents in response to the NHS Plan.* London: RCGP, 2000.

20 Royal College of Nursing, 2000. *Op. cit.*

21 Department of Health. *Improving working lives in the NHS.* London: Department of Health, 1999.

22 Department of Health. *Improving working lives standard: NHS employers committed to improving the working lives of people who work in the NHS.* London: Department of Health, 2000.

23 Smith G, Seccombe I. *Changing times: a survey of registered nurses in 1998.* Brighton: Institute for Employment Studies, 1998.

24 Finlayson B. *et al.*, 2001. In short supply: the extent of the NHS nursing shortage. *Op. cit.*

25 Finlayson B, Dixon J, Meadows S, Blair G. In short supply: the policy response to the shortage of NHS nurses. Submitted for publication, September 2001.

26 *Ibid.*

27 Department of Health. Press release. 13 March 2001.

28 Royal College of Nursing. *RCN response to new fund to address nurse recruitment and retention.* Press release. 13 March 2001.

29 General Practitioners Committee. Golden hellos and golden goodbyes. *GPC News* 2001; 20 July.

30 Smith G, Seccombe I, 1998. *Op. cit.*

31 Finlayson B. *et al.*, 2001. In short supply: the policy response to the shortage of NHS nurses. *Op. cit.*

Valuing our greying workforce

Sandra Meadows and George Blair

INTRODUCTION

The staffing crisis in the NHS is not new. Much government policy is bent around attempting to address these capacity problems in order to improve the quality of care in line with the Plan. A focus on older staff, however, offers a new perspective on solving the problem. This paper examines a workforce that is growing older and more disillusioned, and points up an increasing trend towards early retirement. It argues that a more sensitive and imaginative approach to both preventing older staff from throwing in the towel and leaving work earlier than planned and to recruiting more older people to Health Service posts is needed urgently.

There are no longer armies of young people queuing to join the NHS. Poor pay and conditions, especially among senior nurses, has seen experienced professional staff leaching away.[1] Figures from the Employers Forum on Age,[2] a lobby group aimed at combating ageism at work and whose members include the

NHS Executive, predict that by 2006 there will be 30 per cent fewer women and 26 per cent fewer men aged between 16 and 24 in the NHS workforce than there were in 1986. At the same time, a third of people in the UK aged between 50 and state pension age – 65 years for men and 60 years for women – (2.8 million people) do not work. Working all the way to pension age has rapidly become the exception rather than the norm. Only 37 per cent of men are still working at age 64 compared to 57 per cent in 1979. In addition, male employment rates now start to fall at around 50 (68.3 per cent), rather than from age 55 as in the past. A similar pattern is emerging for those women with occupational pension schemes and significant lengths of service.

Within our health services, older staff are a valuable resource that is very difficult to replace. Not only do they have myriad experience and expertise but, as the population ages, the workforce of the NHS needs to reflect in its age diversity the population that it serves. Many older people find it far easier to relate to staff who are established and who they feel have enough life experience to empathise with their problems. These older staff should not be lost through ageist or other inappropriate personnel practice.

In the light of these statistics, retaining and indeed recruiting older people to the NHS workforce can be seen as good practice and crucial if we are to have the number of skilled practitioners to meet the requirements of the Government's modernisation agenda.

THE AGEING WORKFORCE AND THE STAFFING CRISIS

In today's developed world, people aged 65 and over represent over 14 per cent of the total population. That share will almost double by 2030.[3] This has huge implications for health and social care in that it results in increased demand for services at the same time as the health and social care workforce is itself ageing and the pool of recruits for certain key professions is shrinking. The general trend in the UK economy in recent years has been for an increased rate of early retirement, particularly in white collar employment.[4] The high rate of early retirement from local government employment has led to a situation where retiring early is the 'expectation for local government staff rather than an exception'.[5] Little work has been done on the retirement behaviour of NHS staff but, should a similar trend emerge, given the age profiles of key staff groups the result could be catastrophic. For example, over the next five to ten years the NHS could and probably will lose through retirement many of its most experienced practitioners. In particular, one in five nurses on the professional register is aged 50 years or older.[6] Although current government policy pays substantial attention to the looming staff replacement challenge, scant consideration has been given to determining the professional development and employment needs of the growing number of middle-aged nurses – or to the implications of the ageing nursing workforce for patterns of employment and for attracting back older returners. Moreover, recognition of the need to adequately support improvements in the health of the NHS workforce also has an age dimension.

Nurses who joined the NHS pension scheme before March 1995 have special retirement rights enabling them to retire with full benefits at age 55. In 1997/8, one in ten nurses on the register was beyond the trigger age of 55 and another one in ten was within five years of that age. The level of retirements is projected to grow from around 5500 a year in the late 1990s to over 10,000 a year by the middle of the next decade. As a consequence, in order to maintain the nursing workforce at its current size (which includes 23,000 vacancies in England alone), the number of new registrants entering employment would have to rise from an average of 21,000 a year between 1995 and 2005 to an average of 24,600 between 2005 and 2015. In order to meet this demand, the required level of intakes to pre-registration nurse education would have to rise from around 24,000 in 1997/98 to 31,000 by 2011/12.[7] As these projected intakes are roughly double the size of actual intakes in recent years, it would seem extremely unlikely that the shortfall can be redressed by the number of newly qualified nurses alone.

Managers hoping to narrow the demand and supply gap through altering skill-mix by increasing the number of health care assistants (HCAs) will be no better off. Approximately 15,800 nursing auxiliaries or HCAs were aged 55 or older in 1996.[8] This represents an imminent retirement/ replacement problem of significant magnitude. A major effort will be required just to increase training and recruitment of HCAs to replace retiring auxiliaries let alone encourage substitution of skills.

The primary care workforce is also ageing. A study carried out in Oxfordshire, Berkshire, Buckinghamshire and Northamptonshire found that 25 per cent of GP principals, 30 per cent of practice nurses, 44 per cent of practice managers and 34 per cent of support staff are aged over 50. This figure rises to 50 per cent of single-handed GPs across the four counties.[9] A survey of 1127 GPs aged

over 50 in the North West Region, commissioned by the NHS Executive last year, found that a quarter planned to retire by the age of 59.[10] Changes in the NHS and patient demands were the most frequently cited reasons. If these figures were extrapolated to all GPs in the region, half of those now aged 50 or more will retire by 2002 at the earliest, and by 2005 at the latest. If they stayed on until the age of 65, the Service would not lose them until 2008. When asked what might convince them to stay, some replied that wild horses could not keep them, but 45 per cent indicated they would consider working on if there were part-time opportunities. The Royal College of General Practitioners (RCGP) suggests that you need to train 150 GP registrars to replace 100 people. Women comprise 55 per cent of those in training and 40 per cent of women doctors do not work full time.

The problem of the ageing medical workforce is not confined to GPs. In their evidence to the 1998/99 Doctors and Dentists Review Body, the Department of Health used existing census data to provide indicators about retention of doctors in the NHS.[11]

Data for the period September 1992 to September 1995 suggested that gross wastage from the consultant grade, for reasons including retirement, resignations and secondments, was about 6 per cent in each of these three years. Of this 6 per cent, there was a variation by age, with those doctors under 50 wasting at 2–3 per cent, those aged 50–54 at 3–5 per cent, and those in their late 50s at 6–10 per cent. Early retirements were higher in 1994–95 than in the previous two years. Another source of evidence, the 1987–1997 Hospital and Community Health Services censuses for England,[12] supported the view that early retirements were higher than a decade earlier.

THE IMPLICATIONS OF EARLY RETIREMENT

The implications of the trend towards early retirement, particularly on the grounds of ill health, are highlighted if we examine the number of people leaving on this basis and the costs. Approximately 1 million people are employed in NHS, of which 96 per cent participate in the occupational pension scheme. Of the first 2000 of 5469 applicants from England and Wales who were granted retirement during 1998–9 because of ill health, the following is significant:

- their mean age was 51.6 years and 72 per cent were female
- the commonest reasons for retirement were musculo-skeletal pathology (49 per cent), psychiatric disorders (20 per cent) and cardio-vascular conditions (11 per cent)
- 87 per cent had worked in the NHS for at least ten years
- almost half of those who retired because of musculo-skeletal or psychiatric conditions (43 per cent in both) thought their ill health was caused through work.[13]

Wide variation exists across occupational groups as to the retirement rate. It is estimated that the cohort of 5469 early retirees will cost the NHS Pensions Agency an additional £416 million up to the age of 70 than would have been expected had they retired normally. Two-thirds of the sum will be received by nurses (£180 million) and doctors (£104 million).[14]

RECRUITMENT STRATEGIES

The problem of the ageing workforce, the lack of strategies to recognise this and the knock-on effect of the consequent early retirement is exacerbated by recruitment problems. In medicine, the NHS continues to rely extensively on doctors from overseas – and this despite the existence of established centralised medical workforce planning, a facility not available to other health professions until fairly recently. In 1997, 44 per cent of the 7229 doctors obtaining full registration with the General Medical Council received their undergraduate training outside the UK.[15] Similarly with nursing, the number of overseas nurses coming to the UK has risen by 48 per cent in 12 months. The vacancy level of nurses is estimated at between 9000[16] (NHS Vacancy Survey) and 22,000[17] out of a total NHS nursing, midwifery and health visiting workforce of 330,000. There are also problems in allied health professions, physiotherapy for example, with currently over 600 vacancies.[18]

A number of research studies have looked at the problems of recruitment and retention in the health services across many of the professions. Only a handful has looked at the ageing of the workforce. Policy options which have been effective elsewhere that the NHS could consider include the following:

- Ensuring that the over-50s have the opportunity to update their skills in ways that take into account variations in learning styles, levels of confidence and status within the organisation. In this respect, continuing professional development should widen its traditional focus from enhancing clinical skills to include skills in business and project planning; budgetary control; partnership working with today's well informed, empowered patients; and multidisciplinary team working. These skills should not be seen as frivolous add-ons. Failures in team working can have as disastrous an impact on the quality of patient care as the possibility of serious professional malpractice. And yet there seem to be few systems in place to rigorously appraise our clinicians in these non-professional areas. For older clinicians in particular, failure in these areas leads more frequently to career curtailment than serious professional malpractice and yet its is often difficult for a senior practitioner to admit significant weaknesses in these areas.

- Successive cohorts of older workers complain of increasing pressures and stress in their working lives. Many would welcome the opportunity to carry on working in less pressurised jobs in the same organisation or elsewhere. Instead, many NHS employees face a cliff edge – the high-pressurised job they have always done or nothing. Downshifting can take many forms, from reducing hours, moving to project work, partial retirement, sabbaticals, annual hours contracts, and so on. For example, some older GPs may find coping with the demands of the current large numbers of patients too much. However, they also have significant experience and clinical skills that they have continued to update, and they are only too aware of the health status of the local population. Rather than early retirement being the only option open to them, their expertise could be used by the developing primary care trusts. They could also be available to undertake locum work to ease the burden on other GPs.

- Within occupational health services, developing sensible practices focusing on job design, workload and skills to do the job across the entire workforce

that take account of ageing and its implications. District nurses often leave the profession because of excessive physical strain caused by lifting patients on their own, leading to significant musculo-skeletal problems. More team working across the nursing disciplines may avoid this. With the appropriate support, it should be possible to encourage job integration that allows a transfer of skills from one setting to another and thus enable staff to make a positive choice about staying or ultimately leaving.

- Using the new flexibilities in the NHS pension. The most significant advantage of the flexibilities is that they allow staff to reduce their hours towards the end of their career and also return on an *ad hoc* basis after their retirement without jeopardising their pensions. This allows a whole array of opportunities, from bringing back skilled staff during times of crisis (e.g. winter pressures) to facilitating a reduction in the number of clinical sessions for those approaching retirement so that they can contribute in other key areas, such as education or mentoring.

- Raising the status and increasing the training and development of some of the roles currently considered low status, for example those of health care and social care assistants. These positions could be repackaged with skills and accreditation attached, which may not only retain the current workforce but might also attract those from other industries who still wish to contribute to society, need a continuing income and might welcome the opportunity for further development.

- Learning from organisations that have successfully recruited and retained older people, such as B&Q, which has highlighted the value of employing older people and has reinforced this consistently by using them in their advertisements, giving them a high profile in their stores and celebrating their successes.

BEYOND FAIRNESS

Within the last three years, the Government has launched a code of practice on age diversity in employment, urging employers not to write off people just because of their age.[19] The code was followed up by an NHS circular in August[20] instructing local Health Service employers to carry out a review to ensure their older staff were being treated fairly.[21] While laudable, this entirely misses the point of the problem in the NHS. It is obviously inappropriate for there to be discrimination against older people, but this not the only issue for the ageing workforce. Convincing them to stay beyond their earliest possible retirement date and being motivated and engaged in imaginative and challenging alternatives to the pressurised treadmill existence of their current roles should form the agenda for tackling the problems of the ageing workforce. If the NHS can succeed in retaining its skilled older workforce in this way then it will be better placed to attract older workers from other organisations and those that make up the 2.8 million in the UK aged between 50 and state pension age who do not currently work. Without ensuring the greater contribution of older staff, the ambitious targets of the NHS Plan for the modernisation of our health services are unlikely to be met.

1   Royal College of Nursing. *Making up the difference: a review of the UK nursing labour market in 2000*. London: Royal College of Nursing, 2000.

2   Cabinet Office. *Winning the generation game*. London: Performance and Innovation Unit, 2000.

3   Employers Forum on Age. *Ageism: too costly to ignore*. London: Employers Forum on Age, 2001.

4   Mullan P. *The imaginary time bomb: why an ageing population is not a social problem*. London: Tauris & Co Ltd, 2000.

5   Audit Commission. *Retiring nature: early retirement in local government*. London: Audit Commission, 1997.

6   UKCC. *Annual report*. London: UKCC, 2000.

7   Buchan J. *Carry on nursing: the implications of the ageing nursing workforce for employees and employers*. London: Royal College of Nursing, 1998.

8   *Ibid.*

9   Noakes B, Johnson N. Don't leave me this way. *HSJ* 1999; 109 (5645): 20–22.

10 Mathie T, McKinlay D. *A general practitioner retirement survey in the North West Region*. London: Department of Health, 1999.

11 Pearson C. The true extent of early retirement. *Employing Medical and Dental Staff* 1999; 17: 10–13.

12 *Ibid.*

13 Pattani S *et al*. Who retires early from the NHS because of ill health and what does it cost? *BMJ* 2000; 322 (7280): 208–9.

14 *Ibid.*

15 Dowrie R, Langman M. Staffing of hospitals: future needs; future provision. *BMJ* 1999; 319 (7218): 1193–5.

16 Department of Health. *Vacancies survey, March 2001*. London: Department of Health, 2000.

17 Royal College of Nursing, 2000. *Op. cit.*

18 Department of Health, 2001. *Vacancies survey. Op. cit.*

19 Department for Education and Employment. *Age diversity in employment.* London: Department for Education and Employment, 1998.

20 Department of Health. *Age diversity in employment.* Health Service Circular 1999/182. London: Department of Health, 1999.

21 *Ibid.*

The potential of community hospitals to change the delivery of health care

Sir Cyril Chantler

INTRODUCTION

Things need to be done differently. This is the clear message of the NHS Plan. Advances in science and technology mean that many who would have died now live into old age, though requiring continuing treatment and care. Forty-one per cent of hospital and community health service expenditure is on those aged 65 or more, who comprise 16 per cent of the population.[1] Health services need to be organised to ensure that complex treatments requiring expensive technology and high levels of skill are available when needed, while less complex interventions and care are delivered as economically and conveniently to the patient as possible.

PROVISION

A recent survey identified 471 community hospitals with 18,579 beds in the UK.[2] Surprisingly, the long-term trend is and has been for a steady expansion in community hospitals and beds.[3] In addition, there are 4370 general nursing homes in England with 150,700 beds and 1070 mental homes with 31,800 beds, the latter having risen by 3500 over the last five years. There has been a worrying and dramatic fall in the number of residential and nursing home places, with a loss of 9700 places in the last year. This appears to be due to a combination of factors, such as the rise in property prices, new regulation concerning room sizes and inadequate state-funded support.[4] The private hospital sector contributes 10,800 beds.[5] In contrast, the number of beds in NHS hospitals has continued to fall to 4.1 per 1000 population, or 243,000.[6] The Organisation for Economic Co-operation and Development (OECD) average for hospital beds is around 7 per 1000 population, with the USA under 4 per 1000 population. A recent analysis[7] compared the Kaiser Permanente health plan in California with the NHS; particularly striking is the lower bed-day usage in Kaiser hospitals, at 270 per 1000 population served compared with 1000 bed days per 1000 population in the NHS. The authors believe that this marked difference is due to better planning of hospital admissions with early discharge to home with support, or to community facilities.

The NHS Plan envisages an extra 2100 beds in acute hospitals and a further 5000 in community hospitals or in intermediate care facilities.[8] The extra resources to fund this expansion in intermediate care will total £405 million by 2003/04, with an additional £600 million investment in personal social services that link to intermediate care.

INTERMEDIATE CARE

The definition of intermediate care, given by the Department of Health,[9] is services that meet all the following criteria:

- they are targeted at people who would otherwise face long hospital stays or inappropriate admissions for acute care, residential care, or continuing NHS inpatient care
- the are provided on the basis of comprehensive assessment with an individual care plan for active therapy
- they have a planned outcome to resume living at home
- they are time limited, normally no longer than six weeks
- they involve cross-professional working, with a single assessment framework, shared protocols and single professional records.

A research programme to evaluate intermediate care as a means to promote independence for older people has been established. The impact of intermediate care on hospital acute admissions and length of stay, health and social outcomes, user and carer satisfaction, costs and savings to the NHS and other agencies, and the cost-effectiveness of intermediate care are being investigated.[10]

Intermediate care covers a range of services that help channel admission to an acute care setting through timely therapeutic interventions which aim to divert a physiological crisis or to offer recuperative services at or near a person's own home.[11] A wide range of services can be encompassed within this definition, such as rapid response teams, intensive rehabilitation services, recuperation facilities, arrangements at general practice or social work level to ensure older people receive a one-stop service, and integrated home care teams.[12] Models that have been described include a primary care directorate in an acute district general hospital, a consultant-led service to provide a link between primary and acute care, a nurse-led inpatient facility, and intermediate care for children.[13]

COMMUNITY HOSPITALS

Community hospitals have not just survived the heyday of the district general hospital but are now enjoying a renaissance:[14] though they have generally prospered in the rural environment, their utility in cities is being re-examined;[15] they enjoy public support[16] and can attract funds from outside the NHS;[17] they link well into the intermediate care model for the delivery of services;[18] they can provide a range of services tailored to the needs of the communities that they serve; and the provision of beds, often nurse-led, for respite, rehabilitation, recuperation or acute nursing care can reduce admissions to district general hospitals.[19,20] However, further work is required to improve the efficiency of such units[21] and to ensure that elderly people are not denied access to appropriate technology in specialised units because of their age.[22]

Twenty per cent of all general practitioners in the UK have admitting rights to community hospitals, and consultant outpatient clinics are held in 66 per cent of hospitals. Other services that are provided in some hospitals include minor injury units, day hospitals, physiotherapy, occupational therapy, speech therapy, chiropody and podiatry, inpatient and day surgery, maternity services, and investigations including X-ray and ultrasound, health improvement centres, haematuria clinics, integrated health and social care, and gastroscopy units.[23,24] Community pharmacists can provide a clinical pharmacy service to support the clinical service.[25] The recent commitment to decentralisation within the NHS, with 75 per cent of NHS funding to be in the control of primary care trusts by 2004,[26] may well provide a further stimulus to the development of community hospitals by primary care trusts or care trusts.[27]

Determining what services can and should be provided in community hospitals is not just a matter for clinicians and managers; the population that is to be served needs to be consulted. This consultation should not simply be to ask through a formal consultation process whether they are happy with what is being proposed; rather, the population should be engaged as equal partners from the outset of the planning process. There is the potential to build social capital[28] and to develop management arrangements for the facilities that provide the population with a say in the running of the services. This approach has been adopted by the primary care group for the development of Dulwich Community Hospital in south-east London.[29]

Figure 4 shows the ideas that have emerged so far, but these will no doubt alter as the consultation proceeds and priorities are established. Flexibility in the design of the facilities will be important because the full development will take some years and inevitably needs will change according to social and technological developments and as experience is gained. An important component of the plans is to encourage evaluation at each stage of the process so that lessons can be learned and shared.

A recent report highlighted the problems that exist in the care and support services.[30] The development of community hospitals as both a hub for the provision of services and the hinge between primary and secondary care may have an important role in aiding the integration between care and support services with health and social services, between professionals and volunteers, and in providing training.

INTEGRATION OF HOSPITALS, COMMUNITY SERVICES AND GENERAL PRACTICE

Experience in the USA has demonstrated the importance of integrated care for patients with serious or chronic illnesses,[31,32] and the development of national frameworks in the UK for specific conditions is part of the same process. Herein lies the importance of community hospitals developed by community care trusts. Primary care groups, as constituent parts of trusts, serving populations of 100,000–150,000 people, have the potential to design community hospital facilities to act as the hinge and hub between acute specialised hospitals and general practice. It is finally a question of size.[33] Services need to be provided at the appropriate level as near to, or preferably within, the patient's own home. The provision needs to be efficient, effective and economic[34] and the planning needs to be flexible.[35,36]

Provision of highly skilled, technologically based acute interventions, with added support from fully trained specialists, requires such services, in acute hospitals, to be organised around populations of at least 500,000 people,[37] though such services do not necessarily have to be provided from a single site.[38,39] While people may be prepared to travel some distance for such treatment, there is evidence that they prefer services to be local and readily accessible wherever possible.[40] Many services currently based in district general hospitals can be provided by specialists working with primary care physicians and teams in community settings.[41] Primary care-based emergency centres linked to consortia of general practitioners and telephone advice centres have the potential to reduce the load on accident and emergency departments in acute hospitals. However, close integration with the main A&E department will be essential if appropriate referrals and care in each are to be assured.[42]

Figure 4: Dulwich Community Hospital – an emerging service model

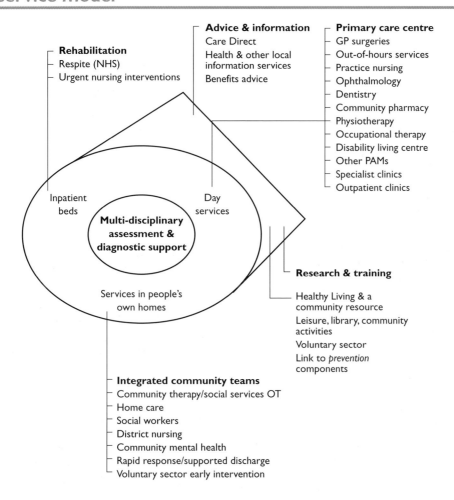

Rehabilitation
Respite (NHS)
Urgent nursing interventions

Advice & information
Care Direct
Health & other local information services
Benefits advice

Primary care centre
GP surgeries
Out-of-hours services
Practice nursing
Ophthalmology
Dentistry
Community pharmacy
Physiotherapy
Occupational therapy
Disability living centre
Other PAMs
Specialist clinics
Outpatient clinics

Inpatient beds

Multi-disciplinary assessment & diagnostic support

Day services

Services in people's own homes

Research & training
Healthy Living & a community resource
Leisure, library, community activities
Voluntary sector
Link to *prevention* components

Integrated community teams
Community therapy/social services OT
Home care
Social workers
District nursing
Community mental health
Rapid response/supported discharge
Voluntary sector early intervention

ROLES AND RESPONSIBILITIES

Integrated care requires teamwork between the specialist and generalist doctors and between all members of the health care team.[43] There is an ever-increasing tendency to specialisation and the introduction of revalidation for doctors, involvement in management and the reduction in time commitment of clinicians will hasten this process. These developments have major implications for the roles and training of doctors. The notion that to be a consultant requires up to seven years of post-specialisation training will need to be re-examined. Revalidation will require doctors to specify what they actually do and demonstrate that they are competent to do it. As technology changes and careers develop, so further training will be required throughout a clinical career. This implies that assessment should be based on competency rather than simply on knowledge. Sufficient time should be available in each doctor's 'job plan' for training and retraining, and that with the actual responsibilities of the work to be undertaken defined, so we should consider the notion of 'just in time' training, rather than long periods of education before undertaking consultant responsibility. Doctors require and receive a broad and deep scientific education in both biomedical science and behavioural science during their undergraduate years. They acquire general experience and further training, during the pre-registration year and as senior house officers. Once they start their specialty training, the task should be to train them in as short a time as possible to achieve the competence necessary to fulfil responsibility either as a principal in practice or as a consultant.

We will also need to consider making it easier for specialists to move to other specialties, again with careful training to ensure competency. The main responsibility of a doctor is to make a diagnosis, and part of this skill comes from involvement in clinical practice.[44] Experienced doctors should be able to 'ladder across' to other specialties without undue restriction from colleges or postgraduate deans, as long as they have demonstrated their competence.

This analysis provokes a further thought. Maybe the time has come to discard the title of 'consultant' and substitute the word 'specialist'. The division of doctors between consultants who work in hospitals and general practitioners who work in the community is peculiarly British and, I would suggest, outmoded. Specialists should work as appropriate in both settings as should generalists. What we should retain is the notion of the generalist as the usual first port of call and the co-ordinator of care.

CONCLUSION

The development of community hospitals and the concepts of intermediate and integrated care have the potential to produce fundamental changes in how treatment and care are provided in the NHS. Flexibility in the design of buildings[45] and in the roles of health professionals, not least doctors, will be needed if this potential is to be realised. It will also require bridging funding to develop the new community facilities, because transfer of funds from secondary facilities to primary care is unrealistic until the new arrangements are in place and have been shown to work.[46]

1 Office of Health Economics. *Compendium of health statistics*. 13th ed. London: Office of Health Economics, 2001.

2 Seamark D, Moore B, Tucker H, Church J, Seamark C. Community hospitals for the new millennium. *British Journal of General Practice* 2001; 51: 125–7.

3 Meads G. Rediscovering community hospitals. Editorial. *British Journal of General Practice* 2001; 51: 91–2.

4 Wheal C. *Are care home owners cashing in on closures? www.society.guardian.co.uk*, 2 May 2001.

5 Department of Health. *Community care statistics 2000*. Bulletin 2001/7. London: Department of Health, 2000.

6 Office of Health Economics, 2001. *Op. cit.*

7 Feachem, Sekhri and White. Personal communication.

8 Secretary of State for Health. *The NHS Plan: a plan for investment; a plan for reform*. Cm 4818-I. London: Stationery Office, 2000.

9 Department of Health. *Intermediate care*. Health service circular 2001/01. London: Department of Health, 2001.

10 Department of Health. *Research to evaluate intermediate care for older people*. London: Department of Health, 2001.

11 Vaughan B, Lathlean J. *Intermediate care: models in practice*. London: King's Fund, 1999.

12 Secretary of State for Health. *The NHS Plan: a plan for investment; a plan for reform*. Cm 4818-I. London: Stationery Office, 2000.

13 Vaughan B, Lathlean J, 1999. *Op. cit.*

14 Meads G, 2001. *Op. cit.*

15 Armstrong D, Baker A H. Health care providers' view about an urban community hospital. *Health and Social Care in the Community* 1997; 5: 347–50.

16 Powell J E. *A new look at medicine and politics*. Tunbridge Wells: Pitman Medical Publishing, 1976.

17 Meads G, 2001. *Op. cit.*

18 Tucker H. Turning community hospitals into assets. In: Meads G, Meads T. *Trust in experience: transferable learning for primary care trusts*. Abingdon: Radcliffe Medical Press, 1996.

19 Hine C, Wood V A, Taylor S, Charny M. Do community hospitals reduce the use of district general hospital inpatient beds? *Journal of the Royal Society of Medicine* 1996; 89: 681–7.

20 Steiner A, Walsh B, Pickering R M, Wiles R, Ward J, Brooking J I, Torgersen D. Therapeutic nursing or unblocking beds? A randomised controlled trial of a post-acute intermediate care unit. *BMJ* 2001; 322: 453–60.

21 Donald I P, Jay T, Linsell J, Foy C. Defining the appropriate use of community hospital beds. *British Journal of General Practice* 2001; 51: 95–100.

22 Grimley Evans J, Tallis R. A new beginning for care for elderly people? *BMJ* 2001; 322: 808–9.

23 Seamark D et al., 2001. *Op. cit.*

24 Tucker, 1996. *Op. cit.*

25 Woolfrey S, Asghar M N, Gray S, Gray A. Can community pharmacists provide a clinical pharmacy service to community hospitals? *Pharmaceutical Journal* 2000; 264: 109–11.

26 Department of Health. *Shifting the balance of power within the NHS: securing delivery*. London: Department of Health, 2001.

27 Meads G, 2001. *Op. cit.*

28 Puttman R. *Making democracy work*. Princeton: Princeton University Press, 1993.

29 *www.dulwichcommunityhospital.nhs.uk*

30 Henwood M. *Future Imperfect? Report of the King's Fund care and support inquiry*. London: King's Fund, 2001.

31 Light D. *An improved NHS: better purchasing and more funds: the 1997 Health Policy Masterclass*. London: Glaxo Wellcome, 1998.

32 Weiner J P, Lewis R, Gillam S. *US managed care and PCTs: lessons to a small island from a lost continent.* London: King's Fund, 2001.

33 Schumacher E F. *Small is beautiful.* London: Bland and Briggs, 1973.

34 Chantler C. National Health Service: the role and education of doctors in the delivery of health care. *Lancet* 1999; 353: 1178–81.

35 Smith R. Reconfiguring acute hospital services. *BMJ* 1999; 319: 797–8.

36 Haycock J, Stanley A, Edwards N, Nicholls R. Changing hospitals. *BMJ* 1999; 319: 1262–4.

37 British Medical Association, Royal College of Physicians, Royal College of Surgeons of England. Joint Working Party. *Provision of acute general hospital services.* London: RCS, 1998.

38 *Ibid.*

39 Posnett J. Is bigger better? Concentration on the provision of secondary care. *BMJ* 1999; 319: 1063–5.

40 Roland M, Holden J, Campbell S. What patients value. In: *Quality assessment for general practice.* Manchester: National Primary Care Development Centre, 1998.

41 Weiner J. *Ibid.*

42 Smith R. How best to organise acute hospital services. *BMJ* 2001; 323: 245–6.

43 Chantler C, 1999. *Op. cit.*

44 Chantler C, 1999. *Op. cit.*

45 Francis S, Glanville R. *Building a 2020 vision: future health care environments.* Medical Architecture Research Unit, South Bank University. London: Stationery Office, 2001.

46 O'Cathain A, Musson G, Munro J. Shifting services from secondary to primary care: stakeholders' views of the barriers. *Journal of Health Services Research and Policy* 1999; 4: 154–60.

Public–private partnerships within health care since the NHS Plan

Anthony Harrison

The term 'public–private partnership' has yet to receive a clear and widely accepted definition. In this article we take a 'broad church' definition, which comprises all the main areas where the NHS interacts with the private sector to ensure that it meets its broad goal of ensuring the universal provision of health care to all residents of the UK.

In doing so, we take a wider view of what should be included than the recent Institute for Public Policy Research (IPPR) report[1] that focused on where private might do what is now public and, therefore, did not ask whether in some areas public might do what is now private. As we shall see in some key areas, a case for that can be made not only in principle but also in practice.

We begin by setting out what the NHS Plan said about private sector involvement and briefly review developments since it was published. We then review developments in the following areas:

- health care services
- drugs
- facilities
- staffing
- R&D
- IT
- support services

We conclude by categorising the main areas of public–private relations and drawing some general conclusions about recent policy developments.

WHAT THE PLAN SAID

The NHS Plan asserts that ideological boundaries or institutional barriers should not stand in the way of better care for NHS patients (para 11.2). Chapter 11 begins with the words:

11.1 The NHS is a huge organisation. Using extra capacity and extra investment from voluntary and private sector providers can benefit NHS patients. The Private Finance Initiative is already delivering new hospitals, on time, to budget as part of the biggest hospital building programme in the history of the NHS. The NHS already spends over £1 billion each year on buying care and specialist services from hospitals, nursing homes and hospices run by private companies and charities. The time has now come for the NHS to engage more constructively with the private sector, and at the same time make more of its own expertise available to employers throughout the country. (p. 96)[2]

But although the NHS already uses private sector facilities extensively, the Plan argues that:

11.5 ... The problem is that most of the arrangements are ad hoc and short term. This way of working provides a poor basis for partnership and value for money. (p. 97)

It went on to announce that, for the first time, there would be a national framework for partnership between the private and voluntary sector and the NHS. This so-called 'Concordat' was intended to provide a better basis for partnership in the provision of care. However, the Plan went on to promote the idea of partnership in three areas not mentioned in the Concordat: pharmaceuticals (para 11.11), research and development (para 11.5), and the provision of premises and facilities management for community health services such as general medical and dental practice and pharmacy (para 4.11). The latter can be seen as an extension of the private finance initiative (PFI) that the Government had already extensively exploited for the provision of hospital facilities and which received further endorsement in the Plan.

Although these references confirm the Government's intention to consolidate and extend the private sector's role within the NHS, its proposals were largely focused on areas where the private sector role was already well established.

Nevertheless, the Plan appeared to indicate a change of direction. That impression was further strengthened by frequent leaks from the IPPR's Commission on Public Private Partnerships in the run-up to the election, which seemed to suggest that the Government was considering a radical change that would mean large-scale privatisation of some parts of the NHS. The Commission had been established in 1999 and, because of its perceived close links with government thinking, the leaks were widely taken as indicative of the direction the Government would take after the election. In the event, the Commission's report[3] was measured rather than radical: although it supported the extension of public private partnerships in principle, that support was accompanied by an effective critique of how they – the private finance initiative (PFI) in particular – had been implemented.

Labour's election Manifesto was also less than radical. It reaffirmed support for the PFI and referred to the possibility that the 'specially built surgical units' might be managed by the private sector and that spare capacity in private hospitals might also be used.

Subsequently, the Prime Minister, in a speech soon after the election,[4] identified four areas where further development of public/private partnership was to be promoted:

So in the NHS: we are using spare capacity in private sector hospitals to perform operations on NHS patients where it makes sense to do so. Second, we will get private sector management to run some of the new stand-alone surgery centres where they offer the best service. Third, we will extend PFI beyond the hospital sector into primary care, social services and the provision of imaging and laboratory equipment. Fourth, we will use private sector management expertise such as in the running of NHS buildings and IT systems.

All of these had largely been anticipated in the Plan and only the second broke new ground. Nevertheless, the trade union movement campaigned through the summer of 2001 against what it saw as a threat of 'privatisation'. In September, the Prime Minister was to have addressed the Trade Union Congress in a bid to defuse the issue. The speech was not in fact delivered due to events in New York and Washington. The text[5] circulated at the time does not go beyond the areas mentioned in the NHS Plan but states the Government's intention to reinforce the regulations bearing on the rights of workers transferred to the private sector.

Neither here nor elsewhere has the Government offered a general rationale for its apparent desire to extend the role of the private sector in the provision of public service. The Prime Minister's speech simply says: 'Where use of the private sector makes sense in the provision of a better public service we will use it. Where it doesn't, we won't.' As we shall see, this pragmatic approach is as likely to lead to an extension of the public role as an expansion of the private.

HEALTH CARE SERVICES

As Justin Keen and colleagues have shown,[6] the private sector is already a substantial contributor to the provision of care. The Plan, however, did not review the full range of the current private sector contribution. Instead, it identified three areas for closer collaboration between public and private sector: elective, critical and intermediate care. In October 2000,

the Department of Health and the Independent Healthcare Association published *For the Benefit of Patients: A Concordat with the Private and Voluntary Health Care Provider Sector*,[7] which set out the terms of this collaboration. The Concordat is described as an enabling framework, designed to leave detailed decisions to be made locally.

> *2.4 Successful partnership will need locally agreed protocols for referral, admission and discharge into and out of NHS and private and voluntary health care provider facilities. There will also be a need for effective agreements on care planning and discharge arrangements with social services departments (this includes determining the most appropriate approach to the development of joint information systems around patient based episodes). (p. 3)*

The three areas mentioned above are discussed in general terms that go little beyond existing arrangements in many parts of the country, and the document's conclusion is exceedingly bland.

> *5.1 Both the Government and the Independent Healthcare Association are committed to continue working together to broaden the aims of the concordat and to look at how the two sectors can work together.*

> *5.2 This can be achieved by the continued development of a long-term relationship at a national level and by ensuring that private and voluntary health care providers are brought into local discussions at an early stage of the planning process. (p. 11)*

The significance of the Concordat therefore stems from the fact that it was published at all, rather than from any specific government commitment.

However, the Plan itself implied that specific developments would take place. The conclusion of Chapter 11 suggests that the key contribution of the private sector lies in reducing waiting times, and in Chapter 4 the Plan proposes the development of elective and diagnostic centres 'to be developed in partnership with the private sector' (para 4.8).

The creation of new elective care and treatment centres in partnership with the private sector potentially implies, as did the terms of the Concordat, a long-term rather than opportunistic relationship. The Plan did not define the terms of the proposed partnership in this area and the Prime Minister, when pressed in the House on the issue, failed to clarify it (see Box 1).

The Plan promised that eight new diagnostic and treatment centres would be available by 2004: a year later than had been increased to 12 and the total from 20 to 29. But, although a number of sites for the new centres were announced in August 2001, it remains unclear how, if at all, they will be different from existing units within NHS hospitals that already specialise in day case treatment and which are effectively isolated from the emergency workload. In particular, the potential for private management to come in and run an NHS facility seems limited and at the time of writing no arrangements of this kind had been announced. Furthermore, in September 2000, BUPA was reported[8] as saying that the amount of work being given to the private sector had fallen since the spring, though overall the numbers being treated were still much higher than in the previous year. In the same month, however, it was announced that a unit was to be established within the Department of Health to promote public–private partnerships that will, among other things, oversee private sector involvement in the new treatment centres.[9]

During the summer of 2001, an entirely new factor came into play. Following a

---

BOX 1: PUBLIC–PRIVATE CONFUSION

The Prime Minister: *As we said in our manifesto, the management of those surgical units could be in the private sector, but those surgical units themselves and their staff will be in the public sector.*

Mr Hague: *No wonder no one knows what the Government is really planning for the National Health Service. The Prime Minister says that there will be privately run surgical units – indeed, that is said in the Labour manifesto – but the Health Secretary says that under no circumstances will any clinical services be run by a private company. Clinical services are one of the things provided by a surgical unit. Being managed is the same thing as being run. The private sector is made up of private companies, so how are those two statements to be reconciled? Will any clinical service be run by a private company?*

The Prime Minister: *We are not privatising clinical services, but what we are saying is that if the private sector can help in the management of those surgical units, the staff, as I have just said, will be employed in the National Health Service, and the distinction is between ensuring that we run and deliver better NHS services and the privatisation of the health service, which is the Conservative party's proposal. (Hansard 2001; 27 June: column 630.)*

decision by the European Court that implied that any patient facing undue delay within their own health care system could be treated free elsewhere in the European Unit, the Government, after initial hesitation, announced that it would after all allow the NHS to use hospital facilities in other EU countries – which might or might be privately owned and operated – to help cut waiting times.

One of the ironies of the current debate is that the general practice contract, a private–public partnership for the delivery of health care services, has been in existence since the foundation of the NHS, along with similar partnerships for dental, optical and pharmacy services. Changes announced in the Plan, as well as policy initiatives taken much earlier, imply that these contractual relationships are no longer satisfactory.

Of these four areas, the most change has occurred within general practice, following the lines already promoted by the Conservative Government in the 1997 NHS Act. The personal medical service (PMS) pilots, for which the Act provided the statutory basis, were introduced to allow the development of new forms of primary care delivery, and these by their nature required new forms of contract that, unlike the old-style contracts, did not leave GPs free to practise as they wished. Although by their nature the pilots embody local variants, they now embody various national requirements including the waiting times targets set out in the Plan for access to a GP or practice staff. The NHS Plan states that the Government expects that, by April 2002, a third of GPs will be working within PMS-style contracts and that the national contract covering all GPs will also be revised so as to embody quality and outcome standards

of the kind contained in PMS contracts. It is clear that in time all GPs will by subject to a more demanding contractual framework as their terms of service are renegotiated.

As far as dentistry is concerned, again there has been considerable change, designed to align the incentives of the individual dentist with the requirements of the NHS as a whole. A series of measures following the announcement in 2000 of the dental strategy[10] have been introduced in an attempt to make good the deficiencies of NHS coverage and also to encourage dental practitioners to maintain and develop their skills. These include:

- *... around fifty Dental Access Centres by March 2001, where patients who are not registered with a dentist can get the full range of NHS dental care. In the year 2001/02 access centres are expected to treat up to half a million patients;*
- *radical new ways for local Health Authorities to improve the availability of NHS dentistry by entering into contracts with NHS Primary Care Trusts, independent organisations or individual dentists; and*
- *better access to urgent out of hours treatment.* (Summary, p. 1)

These measures represent a response to the poor levels of access to NHS dentistry experienced in some parts of the country. In taking them, the Government has acknowledged that the traditional form of contract with the individual independent practitioner can no longer be relied upon to ensure a universal service.

The contractual basis for community pharmacy also looks set to change. A study carried out for the Royal Pharmaceutical Society of Great Britain[11] found that the existing contract, largely unchanged since the foundation of the NHS, had not promoted beneficial changes in practice and was not responsive to the changing environment within which community pharmacists work. More recently, changes to the way that bulk purchases are made of generic drugs, which we consider below, and the development of medicines management will inevitably lead to contractual change.

Medicines management involves the deployment of pharmacists' expertise in processes such as medication reviews and continuing support for patients with chronic conditions. The NHS Pharmacy Plan[12] states that by 2004 all primary care groups and trusts should have such schemes in place.

In the NHS Plan, the Government also announced its intention to create the legal framework that would allow health authorities to test out innovative ways of contracting for pharmacy service and also to change the national framework designed to 'establish minimum standards and to promote and reward high quality services' (para 4.11). In July 2001, the Government announced a series of medicines management pilots designed to improve the general standard of prescribing. The initiative is designed to encourage:

> ... pharmacists [to] work more closely with GPs as part of the primary care team to deliver real improvements to prescribing and healthcare, for example, reviewing the cases of patients with complex medication schemes to check for unfamiliar side effects. (p. 1)

This represents a new role for pharmacists (for which the present contract provides

no incentive) who, in all but extreme circumstances, currently confine their role to executing GPs' (and increasingly nurses') prescribing decisions.

Because most pharmacy services outside hospitals are deeply embedded in the private sector, the process of bringing pharmacists into the NHS fold is unlikely to go as far as it may with doctors and dentists: instead, the nature and content of the pharmacy contract is likely to change radically to take on board the developments reviewed here as well as changes in the supply of generic drugs, which we consider in the following section.

As the examples show, the old-style private contractor relationship is becoming increasingly irrelevant to current requirements. Although only a few GPs and dentists are becoming salaried employees, in effect the changes briefly set out here are moving community practitioners into a relationship that is a contract of employment in all but name.

DRUGS

Since the earliest days of the NHS, there has been a close if at times uneasy relationship between the pharmaceutical industry and the NHS. From the 1950s onwards, the NHS and the industry have been involved in an implicit partnership embodied in the Pharmaceutical Price Regulation Scheme (PPRS).

By and large, the implicit partnership between government and industry has worked to the satisfaction of each side. An assessment by the Health Committee[13] came to the conclusion that the PPRS was slightly tilted towards the interests of the industry but it did not suggest any major revisions: its main recommendation, adopted by the Government, was that the way the agreement worked should be more explicit. The Government subsequently concluded that the scheme should be revised to:

- be more transparent in terms of its operational framework;
- deliver greater compliance than previous PPRS agreements;
- provide greater support to R&D, innovation and competition. (p. 1)

As a result, the Department of Health now publishes an annual report on its workings. The year 2000 report indicates that:

> ... the Government is keen to continue the support for R&D provided by the PPRS and the price paid by the NHS for medicines should include a contribution to the cost of research. To achieve this the 1999 scheme provides a small additional allowance for newer medicines during their patent life. (p. 1)

In early 2000, a Task Force on the Competitiveness of the Pharmaceutical Industry was established (see terms of reference in Box 2 below), which was explicitly aimed at finding ways in which the UK pharmaceutical industry might be supported by public policy.

These terms of reference make it clear that the main focus of the Task Force is the industry rather than the NHS or its users. The main conclusions of the work[14] are in line with this assessment. They are:

- Industry and Government agreed on the essential role that intellectual property rights (IPR) and the TRIPs agreement play, and should continue to play, in the flow of innovative medicines. One of the most important outputs of the Task Force is the renewed industry/Government partnership to work towards improving access to medicines in developing countries.

- Streamlining licensing procedures for essential research involving animals has been agreed, cutting red tape and improving animal welfare. This complements amendments to the Criminal Justice and Police Bill and Malicious Communications Act to tackle harassment and intimidation by animals rights campaigners.

- A more forward looking strategic dialogue about developments in healthcare and the market for medicines in the UK. For example, Government and industry are engaged in comprehensive discussions about how NICE operates, including its impact on the uptake of new medicines, on the competitiveness of the industry, and on the economy more generally. These discussions will inform a review of NICE, including all stakeholders, to be held in July.

- Involving the industry closely in the development of NHS services – such as ensuring the NHS stays at the forefront of development of modern treatments and research, better use of the NHS database for pharmaceutical research and development, improving information to patients, securing better patient involvement in taking medicines and ways of enabling people to secure better access to those medicines not available on the NHS.

- Agreement that new policy measures should not be viewed in isolation, but as part of the overall environment. The impact of new policy directions on UK competitiveness ought to be considered with the pharmaceutical industry prior to implementation.

- Industry and government agreed positions on a range of medicines policy issues

**BOX 2: TASK FORCE ON THE COMPETITIVENESS OF THE
PHARMACEUTICAL INDUSTRY – TERMS OF REFERENCE**

I. *Identify all the criteria for maintaining and developing the competitiveness of the UK as a
successful and effective base for an innovative pharmaceutical industry in a global market.*

II. *Address the following specific issues:*

   1. *Given the role of NICE in relation to judgements about clinical and cost-effectiveness and
other measures intended to improve the quality of prescribing in the NHS, consider how the
home market can best support the international competitiveness of innovative medicines
produced for the home and international market by the R&D industry in the UK.*

   2. *The recognition of intellectual property for pharmaceuticals in the context of:*
- *resolution of the tensions caused by national pricing of medicines and the free movement
of goods within the European Single Market;*
- *global trade in pharmaceuticals.*

   3. *Evaluate the importance of the clinical research infrastructure of the NHS and the benefits
and costs of its use by industry as a location for clinical studies.*

   4. *Consider the aspects of the economic climate in the UK which foster or constrain the
competitiveness of an innovative pharmaceutical industry, and identify any changes which
would significantly strengthen that environment for the industry.*

   5. *Identify further steps that might be taken to foster the development of a vibrant
biopharmaceuticals sector, including examination of the potential for technology clusters to
develop, taking into account the interface with land use planning.*

   6. *Identify the potential for promoting further partnership between the industry and academia
and industry and government.*

   7. *Consider the future development from a competitiveness point of view of the European
medicines licensing system especially in relation to the respective roles of the EMEA and
national agencies.*

III. *Assess, in the light of the Task Force's work, how well the UK is currently meeting the criteria
identified at I above and what further action is needed.*

under discussion in the European Union.
The scope of these has included aspects of
how the EU medicines licensing systems
might develop, issues around EU
enlargement and some key matters of IPR
protection.
- Indicators of performance and
competitiveness have been agreed which
will allow government and industry to
measure and monitor the progress of the
UK as a competitive location for
pharmaceutical investment. (PR
2001/015)

When the report was published, Lord
Hunt acknowledged that there was an
inherent tension between the interests of
the industry and those of the NHS. But
he added:

*The Task Force has shown it is possible to
reconcile these interests in ways that are
mutually beneficial to the industry, to
government, to the NHS and its patients
and to the nation as a whole.* (PR
2001/015)

This remains a hope rather than a firm expectation, since the Task Force report did not in fact set out just how the competing interests were reconciled nor indeed, prices apart, where the areas of potential dispute were – though the first item under the second section of the terms of reference suggests that NICE might be one such.[15]

In one area, relations between government and industry deteriorated significantly. The price of generics does not fall within the scope of the PPRS. Instead the NHS has relied on competition between suppliers and the incentives bearing on community pharmacists to act as efficient purchasers.[16] In August 2000, however, a maximum price scheme was introduced following massive increases in the prices the NHS had to pay for some generic drugs.

This scheme was essentially a short-term measure. The Government subsequently commissioned a review of the generics market from OXERA consultants.[17] This was published in July 2001 along with a discussion paper[18] that, drawing on the OXERA report, put forward two main options for the control of the cost of generic drugs:

- a reform option, which leaves present procurement arrangements intact but changes the basis on which reimbursement prices are calculated. It potentially includes an element of statutory price control; and
- a proposal for the introduction of central purchasing, through competitive tendering, replacing present purchasing arrangement. (p. 4)

The OXERA report itself argues that the price control had not succeeded in effectively containing the cost of generics for several reasons:

- There is a lack of transparency over the nature of the market and prices. Reimbursement prices often differ significantly from true market prices. Price lists in some cases appear to be produced solely for the purpose of satisfying the requirements of the Prescription Pricing Authority (PPA). Prices and the nature of the markets are most opaque to the ultimate payer – the NHS. This is unacceptable.
- The effectiveness of current purchasing and reimbursement arrangements depends on community pharmacies' independence and ability to purchase from whichever supplier can offer them the best deal. Vertical integration has increasingly undermined that independence, weakened the effects of the discount inquiry and further obscured the operation of the market.
- There is evidence that the market for certain generics is concentrated in the hands of just one or two suppliers, increasing the vulnerability of the NHS to shortages in the event of production problems. Overall there is a lack of information on how competitive the market is.
- In addition, the question remains whether present arrangements make the best use of the buying power which the NHS – as the dominant UK customer for such medicines – should be able to exert. (pp. 3–4)

As a result, the NHS was not getting a good 'deal'. Because of the paucity of data, the consultants could not estimate with confidence the extent of overpayment. They therefore made a broad estimate of some £100 million, with a large margin of error round that figure. A further weakness in existing arrangements identified by the consultants is that the market appears to work in such a way that shortages (or perceived shortages) are magnified, leaving the Department of Health struggling to maintain spending within cash limits. In fact, it appeared that the increases experienced in 2000 did not reflect absolute shortages in the supply chain – in the end patients did get the drugs they required – but rather a maldistribution of available supplies, which the reimbursement regime may itself have encouraged.

The OXERA analysis clearly implies that the Department of Health will have to play a larger role in the generics market. At minimum it will have to monitor it more effectively so that the existing regulatory system (if retained) can be better based: it may have to go further and enter the market as the dominant purchaser, thereby replacing the role of (private sector) pharmacists. If OXERA is right in suggesting that vertical integration in the supply and distribution chain is reducing competition (as well as transparency), then the Department of Health will be pushed in the direction of taking active steps to manage the market by, for example, easing the process of licence transfer to promote competition and by taking other measures to promote alternative sources of supply.

FACILITIES

The Autumn 2000 issue of *Health Care UK* reviewed the progress of the private finance initiative in respect of hospital building and concluded that there was little evidence of it making a significant contribution to reducing the costs of hospital services. It also argued that the main focus of the initiative, the acute hospital trust, was misplaced.

The NHS Plan acknowledged this point stating that: 'Where there is a major PFI deal to build a new hospital ... we will, where appropriate, include local NHS primary and intermediate redevelopment too.' In November 2000, the Secretary of State enlarged on this criticism:

> The Health Secretary wants to see PFI extended beyond the hospital gates to include GP surgeries, community pharmacies, health centres, intermediate and long term care facilities. He wants to introduce PFI schemes covering the whole local health service – bringing together improved facilities from the GP to the general hospital.[20]

But, this concession apart, the Government has continued to press ahead with hospital building schemes through the PFI route, more or less as it has done since 1997.

The Plan also announced the Government's intention to enter into new forms of partnership to finance the improvement of primary care premises, the NHS Local Improvement Finance Trust, subsequently known as LIFT.

> ... a new public private partnership within a new equity stake company – the NHS Local Improvement Finance Trust (NHS Lift) – to improve primary care premises in England. The priority will be investment in those parts of the country – such as the inner cities – where primary care services are in most need of expansion. As a result of this NHS Plan:
>
> - up to £1 billion will be invested in primary care facilities
> - up to 3,000 family doctors' premises will be substantially refurbished or replaced by 2004. (para 4.11, p. 45)

LIFT represents an entirely new mechanism aimed at tackling an entirely different problem to the PFI. The low level of investment in hospitals can be attributed simply to a lack of Treasury funding: the organisation and incentives required for new building have been in place. In respect of the funding of primary care premises, both funding and organisation have been missing.

The LIFT prospectus, issued in July 2001, states that investments in primary care premises tend to be made on a piecemeal basis, are not designed to achieve integrated service delivery, and are not concentrated in areas of greatest need and are inflexible. GPs face significant disincentives to practising in inner city areas – too restrictive leases and the risk of negative equity. The standard of existing premises is often poor: access for those with disabilities is often difficult.[21]

In part, these justifications echo those for using the PFI for hospitals – the need to bring about a rapid inflow of capital to modernise an outdated set of capital assets. In part, however, they stem from different considerations: the (presumed) benefits of bringing together different health care professionals and of offering premises on a wider range of terms than now exist.

LIFT is intended to operate at both national and local level. At the national level there is to be a LIFT joint venture company with Partnerships UK. The latter is itself a PPP: it is 51 per cent owned by the private sector and 49 per cent by the Treasury and the Scottish Executive. Its corporate objective is to facilitate the development of PPPs. The process of developing LIFT is still underway and, despite the fact that it appears to be the Government's chosen

instrument, a number of questions remain as to how it is intended to operate.

As the IPPR report points out (p. 144), these arrangements look likely to lead to confusion about who is responsible for what, and there is also a risk that, as with the PFI, it will appear to be the only game in town. Furthermore, the nature of the local company format means that the local NHS will be tied in to one partner for an indefinite period, a situation that could too easily encourage inefficiency. It is also hard to see how competing public and private interests will be reconciled within the proposed company format. Although the intention is that public and private interests will be represented on it, it is not clear how stable such arrangements will be over time since local LIFT company share will be tradeable, opening up the possibility that local involvement may cease at some future time.

STAFFING

The NHS uses short-term contract staff to maintain cover when full-time staff are on leave and to meet peaks in demands. Many trusts operate their own banks, others rely on the private sector. In February 2001, the Executive issued *NHS Professionals*,[22] which is designed to:

> ... set the standards for in-house NHS agency arrangements and will in time provide a nation-wide service offering Trusts cost-effective, flexible access to the services of healthcare staff across the full range of clinical and support skills. It will complement and build upon the existing 'bank' and temporary staffing arrangements through the expansion of bank operations via collaboration between NHS organisations within local labour markets.

BOX 3: PUBLIC–PRIVATE PARTNERSHIP IN RESEARCH

Since the Task Force report was published, the Manufacturing Molecules Initiative was launched by the Science and Innovation Minister. This is to designed to provide funding for:

- *new technology to produce better drugs to tackle killer diseases like heart disease and cancer;*
- *new technologies to produce ingredients for drugs in the pharmaceutical industry more quickly and efficiently;*
- *projects using 'green chemical technology' – new environmentally friendly ways of working and ways of reducing the potential hazard to workers and the general public from chemicals and their by-products.*[19]

Although NHS Professionals is not specifically designed to eliminate the private sector role, that is the clear implication of its successful development. Indeed, in announcing in September that the scheme was up and running, Health Minister John Hutton said that 'the NHS will no longer have to rely exclusively on commercial recruitment firms for temporary staff ... ensuring better value for money'.[23]

R&D

In the previous issue of *Health Care UK*, we described the contribution of the private/voluntary sector and the public sector to health-related R&D. The outstanding feature of the current situation is the dominance of the private sector which, as noted above, is explicitly allowed for in the determination of the terms of the PPRS. Despite this dominance, the private sector is nevertheless highly dependent on the NHS, both for the execution of research supported by commercial research grants and for the use of the NHS as a 'test bed' for its products and particularly clinical trials.

The Plan's discussion of R&D is very limited and is confined to aspirations of a general nature:

11.15 Working with the private sector and other partners we will commission NHS research and developments in new centres of excellence. These medical knowledge parks will evaluate all aspects of the emerging developments in genetics, from the laboratory testing to the requirement for counselling of patients. They will bring together NHS research, the private and charitable sectors alongside front-line NHS staff and patients. (p. 99)

Neither the Plan nor the Task Force is explicit about the nature of the partnership that is envisaged. However, evidence presented to the House of Commons Science and Technology Committee,[24] in the course of its investigation of cancer research, indicated that the terms of the existing partnership were not clear. The Committee concluded that 'if the pharmaceutical industry is to be encouraged to do more cancer clinical trials in this country the costs of doing so must be made competitive with those in other countries'. (p. 14)

The Task Force also considered this issue, reporting that:

6.15 Surveys across many companies suggest that between 1993 and 1998, the costs of Phase II-III clinical research in the UK increased by 50%. Compared with our close European partners, the UK is more expensive and the gap appears to be widening.

Its report indicates that the Government intends to tackle this particular area and also to define more generally the nature of the public–private partnership:

6.29 The Department of Health will review its guidance on the relationship between prices charged by the NHS and the cost of studies with the intention of improving the transparency and consistency of pricing. The review will be informed by evidence of variations in NHS approaches to pricing and the cost to industry of conducting its research in other major markets. The overall aim will be, within the constraints of EC law and Government policy for public services, to minimise impediments to the UK's competitiveness for clinical trials when compared with major EU and North American markets. This review will be completed by 30/06/01. (p. 62)

It goes on:

6.31 A Research Partnership Agreement is to be drawn up between the UK pharmaceutical industry represented by the ABPI and the Department of Health/NHS, that acts as a framework for continued interaction. It will parallel that for non-commercial (charity) funded research (this to cover issues of mutual interest and arrangements for collaborative work, funding, timeliness, communication between companies and NHS bodies and the quality of research in the wider public interest). Following the development of a Research Partnership agreement, Industry and Government will establish a formal mechanism to continue discussion. (p. 62)

At the time of writing, the terms of this partnership had not appeared.

In a separate stream of development, originating in the DTI, a process known as Foresight began in the early 1990s that attempted to define areas of opportunity for UK industry. In respect of health, programmes were established, focusing on ageing and health and diet.

A 1995 report[25] had argued that pressures within the pharmaceutical industry would tend to mean that certain areas of health need would be neglected but that, nevertheless, the relationship between business and government would of necessity become closer, because of their joint interest in medicine assessment. The 2001 report Healthcare 2020[26] emphasises that drugs and medical equipment development is inherently a 'partnership' in which public and private interests are necessarily intermingled. It therefore sets out a number of areas where it believes private–public interaction would be useful, including measures to improve knowledge transfer and exchange of personnel. But perhaps the key point it makes is that the NHS should develop a proactive stance with regard to innovation, rather than being a passive recipient of innovations from the private sector and that effective non-commercial testing facilities should be developed to improve the commercial development process. If this is right, it would lead to expansion of the NHS role both as an informed purchaser and as a nursemaid of innovation, particularly in those sectors such as equipment and devices, where small firms are often the source of innovation but often do not have the resources to develop and market new products effectively.

IT

The Plan sets out very briefly some of the elements of the IT strategy published as a separate document.[27] These include:

- *an extra £250 million invested in information technology in 2003/04*
- *electronic booking of appointments for patient treatment by 2005*
- *access to electronic personal medical records for patients by 2004. By then 75% of hospitals and 50% of primary and community trusts will have implemented electronic patient record systems*
- *electronic prescribing of medicines by 2004 giving patients faster and safer prescribing as well as easier access to repeat prescriptions*
- *all GP practices will be connected to NHSnet by 2002, giving patients improved diagnosis, information and referral*
- *through investment in electronic patient records all local health services will have facilities for telemedicine by 2005 allowing patients to connect with staff electronically for advice.* (pp. 48–49)

The Plan does not refer to the private sector. However, IT projects had been commissioned through the PFI route – sometimes as part of a hospital scheme and sometimes as free-standing contracts, while the private sector was already playing a key role in relation to NHSnet through contracts with BT, BT Syntegra and Cable & Wireless.

In respect of NHS Direct, in September 2000 a seven-year partnership with Axa Assistance to provide clinical decision support system for NHS Direct was announced. This agreement meant that Axa Assistance became the sole provider of clinical support decision systems to the NHS (in the early days of NHS Direct, three systems were used). In return, however, the NHS will have total control over the development of the system, which will be known as the NHS Nurse Clinical Assessment System, and the NHS will receive up to 20 per cent of all overseas sales revenues over the life of the contract.

As far as IT projects in general were concerned, procurement experience had not been happy. Accordingly, a review of IM&T procurement was announced in *Information for Health*. The resulting report,[28] published in June 2000, set out a wide range of procedures for national and local projects: however, the general nature of the relationship with the private sector was not discussed.

The revised information strategy,[29] published in January 2001, refers to the fact that the existing contracts for NHSnet expire around 2003 and will have to be negotiated, and also declares the intention of procuring a new national payroll and human resources system from the private sector. It also seems clear that the IT support for the patient record system will be financed through a PFI deal.

Unlike the supply of hospital facilities, the private sector role has inspired little controversy or debate. Instead, the main focus has been on implementing a nationally determined strategy.

As noted already, the Prime Minister indicated in his July speech that contracts may be let for the supply and management of IT facilities. There has been no indication that the difficulties experienced with IT contracts in other parts of the public sector[30] have led to any change of mind about the suitability of IT provision for complex and long-term contracts.

SUPPORT SERVICES

From the early 1980s onwards, some NHS support services have been subject to competitive tendering, while, from the *Competing for Quality* White Paper[31] onwards, the NHS was encouraged to increase the range of services bought from the private sector. The financial pressures to which trusts were subject during this period, including the requirement for annual cash-releasing efficiency gains, meant that most did. With the 1997 White Paper,[32] the emphasis changed: competitive tendering for these services was downplayed,[33] but it was not until the Plan itself that something was put in its place. This was a less directive approach known as Best Value (see Box 4).

Best Value was originally introduced into local government as a response to the perceived failures of the competitive tendering regime introduced by the Conservatives. There is now substantial experience of its operation. A discussion paper from the Improvement and Development Agency (IDEA) argued that, though Best Value had produced service improvements, it risked getting bogged down in procedures.[34] A subsequent report from the Audit Commission[35] suggested that 'the Government should take stock'. Many councils, it found, were yet to come to grips with the most challenging aspects of Best Value.

It remains unclear precisely how it will work within the NHS. What is clear, however, is that the Best Value approach rests on the ability of the public sector to reform itself – albeit supported by some, as yet unspecified, inspection process.[36]

BOX 4: BEST VALUE

The duty of Best Value:
To deliver services to clear standards covering both cost and quality, by the most effective, economic and efficient means available. It came into force on 1 April 2000 and applies to all local government services, including social services.

The aim of the Best Value process:
To secure continuous improvements in performance, and to deliver services that bear comparison with the best. Councils are expected to demonstrate that they have taken into account the four 'Cs' – Challenge, Compare, Consult & Compete.

What processes are involved?
All councils must ensure that their services are responsive to the needs of citizens, are efficient and of high quality and provided within a clear policy framework. They must prepare annual Best Value Performance Plans, setting out their strategic objectives and corporate priorities. Over a five-year period they must review all their services to consider new approaches to service delivery and set demanding performance targets that will deliver continuous improvement. There are also new powers for central Government to intervene in authorities that are failing to deliver Best Value.

Full details can be found on www.local-regions.detr.gov.uk/bestvalue

OVERVIEW

The range of public–private relationships may be grouped as follows:

- contracts between the NHS and the private sector for supply of clinical and support services
- less formally defined relationships, some of a quasi-regulatory nature
- joint ventures.

Most of the areas we have reviewed fall into the first group. Here, three different trends are apparent. First, a switch to long-term contracts for the supply of long-life assets, particularly important for the provision of hospital services. Prior to the introduction of the private finance initiative, the private sector was already the main supplier of all the elements involved in hospital provision (and in some, such as construction, the sole supplier): hence, the main innovation is not in the use of the private sector but rather in the precise nature of the contractual arrangements. Second, a move towards the redefinition and tighter specification of existing long-term contracts for the delivery of care in community settings. Although there are only limited signs so far, this trend may result in full integration of community professionals into NHS employment. Third, a retraction from a blanket commitment to open up support services to competitive tendering towards a case-by-case approach.

The Concordat falls into the second group. It does not represent a contract, but rather an attempt to define mutually beneficial behaviour, including some areas such as training that fall outside the day-to-day process of supplying care. A related development has been the introduction of a regulatory regime for the private sector paralleling that in the public sector.[37]

Development of drugs and its supporting R&D also falls into the second group. Here, the main trend is towards greater explicitness about the roles of the public and private sectors and where their interests lie. The Task Force can be seen as an attempt to identify where public action can support private. But in the generics field, the implication of the developments recorded above is that the public sector has to expand its role to displace what are now private sector functions, albeit carried out in part for the benefit of the public.

The third group is currently very small: it comprises the arrangements for the marketing and development of the software used for NHS Direct and the quite different set of arrangements proposed for the development of community health care facilities. Here, there is little experience to go on, but the main question this development raises, as noted above, is whether it is possible to harmonise the interests of the public and private sectors within the one agency or agreement.

As this brief survey has shown, neither the Plan nor the Prime Minister's statement was comprehensive, nor were either based on any explicit analysis of those situations where the private sector could be expected to perform better than the public. In many of the areas considered above, there has been very little public debate and still less evidence or argument for the developments described or the specific form they have taken, or whether the benefits claimed for private action could be obtained by the public if its procedures were changed.

However, in two areas a rather different conclusion could be reached. In respect of generic medicines and to a lesser extent pharmaceuticals more generally, the

Government has begun to study in detail the way that existing relationships work and how they might be improved. In the case of generics, that will almost certainly lead in the direction of the Department of Health becoming more interventionist in the market for manufacturing and supplying drugs and, if the second of the two options put forward is chosen, it will expand its role by taking over the purchasing function from community pharmacists. In respect of drugs more generally, the Government has so far appeared content to work within the framework of the PPRS, but the work of the Task Force and the Foresight Health Panel suggests that improvements in drug development depends as much on the public (or non-commercial sector such as universities) developing its role as an extension of the private sector.

These analytic developments are in sharp contrast to the developments in respect of facilities, particularly the LIFT proposals. The latter appear to rest on no understanding of local markets for such facilities, nor is it underpinned by any analysis of why the current arrangements, which are largely the responsibility either of the private sector or of self-employed professionals, do not work. Furthermore, the LIFT prospectus offers no means of measuring whether the proposed arrangements offer value for money nor how, where there is conflict, public and private interests will be reconciled. In this area, the Government appears intent on forging ahead – as it has done with the private finance initiative in respect of hospital building – without serious consideration of the alternatives.

As far as PPPs are concerned, the IPPR has, as noted above, done some of its thinking in public for them. However the Commission report,[38] published in June 2001 but after the election, took a far more considered and balanced approach than the leaked reports had suggested. Indeed, instead of urging that the Government press ahead with more private involvement, it instead embodied a plea for 'open-mindedness'. Its recommendations represent a very cautious piecemeal approach to the extension of the private sector's role (see Box 5).

BOX 5: IPPR RECOMMENDATIONS

Purchasers should take a case-by-case approach towards assessing the package of services that are included within a PPP.

A partnership approach may be appropriate if the following criteria are satisfied:

- *service outcomes can be clearly specified and measured*
- *value-for-money can be demonstrated – indicating that transaction costs and costs of monitoring the contract are offset by efficiency gains*
- *clear purchaser–provider relations exist*
- *contract terms do now allow scope for the provider to select only the most 'profitable' clients*
- *an integrated service can be provided, with close working and clear communication between providers*
- *providers demonstrate an appropriate public service ethos.* (p. 37)

Our analysis suggests a rather different if complementary conclusion: that the emphasis should be as much on private sector failure and the potential for public intervention to improve it. This emphasis has become unfashionable but, as some of the examples given above indicate, particularly for drugs and R&D, the Government will, in some cases, be pushed in that direction.

1 Institute for Public Policy Research. *Building better partnerships: the final report of the Commission on Public Private Partnerships.* London: IPPR, 2001.

2 Secretary of State for Health. *The NHS Plan: a plan for investment; a plan for reform.* Cm 4818-I. London: Stationery Office, 2000.

3 Institute for Public Policy Research, 2001. *Op. cit.*

4 Prime Minister. *Public service reform.* Speech at the Royal Free Hospital, 16 July 2001.

5 Prime Minister. Speech at the Trade Union Congress, 11 September 2001.

6 Keen J, Mays N, Light D. *Public–private partnerships.* London: King's Fund, 2001.

7 Department of Health and the Independent Healthcare Association. *For the benefit of patients: a concordat with the private and voluntary health care provider sector.* London: Stationery Office, 2000.

8 BUPA rues missed summer window. *HSJ* 2001; 111 (5771): 6.

9 New unit promotes private sector in NHS. *Financial Times* 2001; 19 September: 7.

10 Department of Health. *Modernising NHS dentistry: implementing the NHS Plan.* London: Stationery Office, 2001.

11 Royal Pharmaceutical Society of Great Britain. *Medicines, pharmacy and the NHS.* London: RPS, 1999.

12 Department of Health. *Pharmacy in the future: implementing the NHS Plan.* London: Stationery Office, 2000.

13 House of Commons Health Committee. *Pharmaceutical Price Regulation Scheme: fourth report to Parliament.* London: Stationery Office, 2000.

14 *www.doh.gov.uk/drugs*

15 The industry was very critical of the early decisions of NICE, which threatened to reduce the market for its products within the NHS.

16 Pharmacists are reimbursed for the medicines they dispense at a standard rate: if they can buy more cheaply by shopping around they can 'pocket' the difference, subject to a claw-back regime.

17 Oxford Economic Research Associates (OXERA). *Fundamental review of the generics medicine market.* Oxford: OXERA, 2001.

18 Department of Health. *Options for the future supply and reimbursement of generic medicines for the NHS: a discussion paper.* London: Stationery Office, 2001.

19 Department of Trade and Industry. *Quicker, better drugs to tackle diseases.* PR/2001/410. London: Department of Trade and Industry, 2001.

20 Department of Health. *More PFI hospitals to provide more NHS beds.* PR 2000/0658. London: Department of Health, 2000.

21 The Department has given the go-ahead for schemes to be developed in six areas: Newcastle, Barnsley, Manchester Salford and Trafford, Camden and Islington, and East London. As this list suggests, the intention is to focus initially on inner city areas, but that emphasis may shift in time.

22 Department of Health. *NHS professionals: flexible organisations, flexible staff.* HSC 2001/02. London: Department of Health, 2001.

23 Department of Health. *NHS staff agency will be operational across the country within a few weeks.* PR 2001/0404. London: Department of Health, 2001.

24 House of Commons Science and Technology Committee. *Cancer research: a fresh look.* London: Stationery Office, 2000.

25 Department of Trade and Industry. Foresight Programme. *Health and life sciences.* London: Department of Trade and Industry, 1995.

26 Department of Trade and Industry. *Healthcare 2020.* London: Department of Trade and Industry, 2000.

27 Department of Health. *Information for health: an information strategy for the NHS 1998–2005: a national strategy for local implementation.* London: Stationery Office, 1998.

28 Department of Health. *NHS IM&T procurement review.* London: Stationery Office, 2000.

29 Department of Health. *Building the information core: implementing the NHS Plan.* London: Department of Health, 2001.

30 House of Commons Committee of Public Accounts. *Forty-first report. The prime project: the transfer of the Department of Social Security estate to the private sector – report together with the proceedings of the committee relating to the report, the minutes of evidence and an appendix.* London: Stationery Office, 1999.

31 Department of Health. *Competing for quality: market testing and reporting.* White Paper. Leeds: Department of Health, 1993.

32 Secretary of State for Health. *The new NHS: modern, dependable.* London: Stationery Office, 1997.

33 According to the Secretary of State when announcing the (re)introduction of matrons in 2001, compulsory competitive tendering 'had failed to drive up standards'.

34 See *www.idea.gov.uk*

35 Audit Commission. *Changing gear.* London: Stationery Office, 2001.

36 Best Value has not yet been applied to central government, but in 2001 it was announced that the roles of the NHS Pensions Agency and NHS Estates would be development in conjunction with private sector partners.

37 Through, in particular, establishment of the National Care Standards Commission.

38 Institute for Public Policy Research, 2001. *Op. cit.*

After the NHS Plan, what next?

Nicholas Timmins

It is less than 18 months since the National Health Service Plan was published – and still less than two years since the Prime Minister declared his aim, later rapidly downgraded to an ambition, to raise health spending in the UK to the European average.

But already the first key dates in the Plan – the host of improvements in shorter waiting times, medical and nursing staff numbers, and more NHS buildings and equipment promised for 2004 and 2005 – feel to be just around the corner.

Already the question is being asked: what happens if the Plan fails? This is not easy to answer, not least because neither success nor failure is easy to define.

The Government will no doubt seek to define success by whether it hits the myriad targets it has set. But it knows the real question will not be whether they are achieved, or appear to have been achieved, but whether the electorate believes that the NHS feels significantly better and that it is still improving.

Whether that will be the case cannot yet be judged. What can be said with some conviction is that the Service will not by then be perfect. After all, even the Government describes its plans for the NHS as a ten-year programme. Some of its most ambitious targets stretch out to 2008 and beyond. And, while there is plenty of room for argument about whether the UK actually needs European ratios of doctors to patients, or patients to scanners, or similar expenditure per head (after all, there is a good case that France and Germany are over-doctored and over-resourced), there is little doubt that the UK's health system has become under-doctored and under-resourced for a rich industrialised country at the start of the twenty-first century.

The Government has, it is true, brought about large increases in training places for doctors, nurses and other therapists. But the sheer time needed to train doctors or to produce experienced nurses means that the impact of these measures will still barely be felt three to four years from now. Given the amounts of money being spent, the NHS is almost bound to feel better. But continued shortages of key staff are likely to mean that it will still feel as though it is struggling.

If the project is not judged a success, however, what then happens? Inevitably, the question of how the NHS is funded will once again come into focus. For, politically, one of the interesting aspects of the Government's decision last year to provide a genuine step change in NHS funding – 6 per cent a year in real terms over four years against the long-run historical average of 3 per cent – is that it failed to silence the debate about alternative ways of funding health care in the UK.

It is not just that bodies such as Civitas, the free market social think-tank spun out of the Institute for Economic Affairs, and the Institute of Directors, or some of the health insurers have continued to sponsor studies and argue the case for a change of funding. These might be described as 'the usual suspects'. Rather, it is that others have stayed with the argument – the Social Market Foundation and the left-of-centre Institute for Public Policy Research, for example.

Equally, government itself now has a Treasury-sponsored study underway into the likely future level of demand for health care and its implications for NHS funding levels. Ostensibly, this work does not enter the area of *how* the NHS should be funded. But, depending on the answers it produces, it may yet lead to that.

This means that those who still believe that a tax-funded, largely free-at-the-point-of-use approach remains the best way to provide health care need to start marshalling their arguments now. But they need to do so in two ways: first, to defend the case; and second, to then work out what would be the best alternative if that case is lost – if, in effect, it becomes politically untenable regardless of the weight of evidence in its favour.

Defending the *status quo* may take some doing. Some of the old arguments will wash much less well in two or three years' time. The argument, for example, that the NHS is cheap and cheerful but works reasonably well will be a lot less convincing when spending is nearer the EU average (however defined) than it is now.

Some arguments will still stand. For example, that the NHS, in comparison with both public and private insurance systems, remains cheap to administer. Equally, tax funding remains re-distributive. And the maintenance of a monopoly purchaser also almost certainly helps restrain health care costs. But the case will need to be remade.

Another element that clearly appeals to the Government is that the NHS keeps employment costs low. Since New Labour came to power, it is clear that both main parties are now committed to what might be called the 'Anglo-American employment model', rather than the social insurance model of much of continental Europe. The aim of both parties now is to keep the costs of job creation low by not loading employers with the cost of health care or pension provision, preferring to provide these services either through individuals' contributions or general taxation. That makes it unlikely that the Government would want to move to a social insurance model for the NHS, not least because employers in France and Germany are increasingly complaining about the costs that it loads onto them.

That, however, runs the risk that alternatives will tend to focus on more individualised private insurance, or voluntary employer insurance, as in the United States – a model to which no one in their right mind would voluntarily head.

In practice, health care systems around the world tend to be shaped by their own particular histories, and transferring models from one country to another has rarely proved easy. But before the crunch comes – possibly as early as 2004 – those who wish to defend the NHS's key goals –

inequity favouring the poor in funding terms, and treatment according to need not ability to pay – need to think not just how to defend the current model but how it might be amended to achieve those aims by different means.

There may be more time than this scenario suggests. Next summer, there will be another comprehensive spending review. Prior to 11 September, it was a reasonable assumption that this would lead to further continued high levels of growth in NHS spending. Given the profound uncertainty at present about the world economic outlook, that can no longer be taken for granted. But some attempt to maintain higher growth levels remains likely, not least because the cash injections currently planned will not, on current trends, take health care spending in the UK to the Prime Minister's target of the European average. In practice, given the time lag that it takes to produce OECD data, no one will know for sure in 2004/05 quite where the UK does stand in relation to the rest of Europe – the most recent data likely to be available will relate only to 2002 or 2003. And, given the depth of the Government's commitment in Chapter 3 of the NHS Plan to the current NHS model, it is hard to see it changing its stance before the next election. Thereafter, however, if the gap between performance and expectation remains unchanged, anything could happen.

The first moves on Labour's side might well be within the general model of tax funding – a move, or partial move, towards hypothecated or earmarked taxes for the NHS, or possibly even a shift to regional organisation for the NHS and a degree of regional funding. But, if the NHS Plan is perceived to have failed, such changes will look more like prevarication than a long-term solution. On the Conservative side, it is too early to judge what a party led by Iain Duncan Smith will support. But it is a fair bet that it will seek some greater use of the private insurance market, whether through tax breaks for employers who provide health cover or tax breaks for individuals.

Either way, by the time of the next election, a much more serious debate is likely to be raging about whether the NHS should remain what it is – a tax-funded, largely free-at-the-point-of-use service. And those who believe in the NHS's values need to give some serious thought to how they could be achieved through some other funding mechanism: one that does not offer only a 'core' service; does not perpetuate, more than the current model does, better care for the better off; and does not turn out to cost a whole lot more for not much real gain in health care.

Of course, the NHS Plan may work – with its targets met and public satisfaction high – and such thought may prove unnecessary. It would not be wise to bet on it.

The NHS: where has all the new money gone?

John Appleby, Chris Deeming and Anthony Harrison

INTRODUCTION

To many looking at the NHS from the outside – and even to many on the inside – there seems to be a mismatch between the huge sums of extra money pouring into the Service and an apparent continued need to make savings. What's going on? Where is all the extra money going?

Just over a year ago, during a Sunday morning TV interview, the Prime Minister pledged to raise total health care spending to match the average of EU countries. And now the new money has started to flow into the system – an 8.9 per cent real terms funding increase in England for this year and around 5 to 7 per cent planned for the next three years.[1]

These increases are unprecedented. Historically, NHS funding increases have averaged around 3 per cent per annum in real terms – that is, after allowing for general inflation in the economy as a whole as measured by the GDP deflator. No one, including the Government, doubts that the NHS needs more money if it is to begin to match the demands and expectations we are placing upon it, but how is all this extra money actually being spent?

A BLUEPRINT FOR SPENDING

The NHS Plan[2] provided a broad indication of where the money should go – more doctors, nurses, equipment and facilities. It also set out a plethora of targets for improvement in the care that patients receive, for example reductions in maximum waiting times both for outpatient appointments and for subsequent treatment. The message from ministers was clear: we've done our bit by finding more money, now you've got to do your's by improving standards.

But the Plan was very thin on financial detail. It did not set out how much all the extra staff and facilities are expected to cost, how much of the increased spending is expected to go on particular service areas or how much extra simply to maintain the existing level of services.

The Government's *quid pro quo* for the extra money has been reinforced through the use of centrally allocated funds – the Centrally Funded Initiatives, Services and Special Allocations (CFISSA) budget of nearly £5.9 billion and the Health Modernisation Fund of £2.2 billion for this year.[3,4] These top-sliced funds are distributed in various ways – some as part of health authorities' unified allocations and some through bidding processes.

The Government's intention is to limit the ring-fencing or earmarking of resources in response to concerns from the NHS.[5] Therefore, it has refrained from ring-fencing all Modernisation Fund monies distributed to health authorities as part of their unified allocations. Nonetheless, it is keen to see that key spending review commitments are delivered and has therefore 'hypothecated' some of the Fund – around £1.1 billion for 2001/02.[6] Hypothecated funds are those that are included in allocations, with the intention that they be spent on the purpose for which they are allocated. This money is in effect tied down to specific services – broadly, the Government's priorities for heart disease, cancer and mental health. Table 1 gives hypothecated funding for 2001/02).

For a typical local health purchaser and its service providers, room for financial manoeuvre has become somewhat limited – on the one hand, historically unprecedented amounts of cash: on the other, equally unprecedented levels of central direction as to its use.

Nevertheless, health organisations have some discretion over the spend of this new money within the broad parameters set by the Department of Health. But what is the level of discretion, and how is it being used?

HOW IS THE NEW MONEY BEING USED?

The bulk of funding for local health services is piped to health authorities through a single unified allocation (the baseline or initial budget). In addition, they will access funding through CFISSA and the Modernisation Fund. So how is all this extra funding being used?

A health authority that has received an additional £100 million on top of its initial budget allocation for this year would find that around half of this increase is linked to government initiatives outlined in the NHS Plan – ring-fenced funds from its Modernisation Fund for coronary heart disease services, smoking cessation services, teenage pregnancy services and disposable tonsillectomy instruments, as well as consultant distinction awards. Health organisations have little or no discretion over the application of these funds.

Table 1: Hypothecated funds for 2001/02[7]

Priority	£m
Cancer and coronary heart disease	450
Waiting times and access	423
Intermediate care and community equipment	188
Information management and technology	113

The remainder of the increase is not tied in this way. But, although the authority enjoys discretion over how this new money is spent, it also has many unavoidable financial commitments. The most important of these are increases in NHS staff pay and prices. Our analysis suggests that this NHS-specific inflation accounts for nearly a third of a typical health purchaser's additional allocations (see Figure 1) – equivalent to around 6 per cent, which is nearly treble the general inflation measure (the GDP deflator) used by government to calculate real spending levels.

Further unavoidable commitments or 'must-dos' approved by regional offices include reducing waiting times for hospital treatment and funds for winter planning. Other funding is set aside for meeting the extra costs of NICE guidelines, PFI payments, and meeting the extra costs of the EU working times Directive. In addition, some funds are clawed back by the Department of Health to cover such things as medical negligence claims.

The NHS is also, for the time being at least, carrying a financial legacy of accumulated debt – effectively the Service has in the past borrowed from the future, and now it is having to pay back. The National Audit Office published accounts of NHS financial performance for 1999/2000 showed that just over half of the 99 health authorities in England and over a third of the 377 hospitals reported a deficit – giving a total overspend of £129 million in England.[7] So what does all this mean?

INFINITE DEMANDS, FINITE MEANS

There is no doubt that a significant chunk of the extra money is buying better and expanded services; patients *are* benefiting from the extra resources. But it is also likely that many services – particularly those not identified as priorities by the Government – are not receiving much of the additional funding (though the staff delivering these services are now, in the main, better paid). Keeping such services going – and in particular dealing with extra demands – is proving difficult given the 'must-dos'.

Figure 1: Where the extra money is going

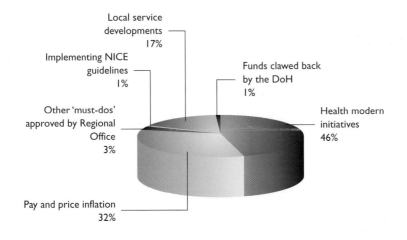

Local service developments 17%

Implementing NICE guidelines 1%

Funds clawed back by the DoH 1%

Other 'must-dos' approved by Regional Office 3%

Health modern initiatives 46%

Pay and price inflation 32%

Moreover, the NHS will continue to struggle to keep up with the additional demands that are placed upon it despite all this extra money. In fact, the improvements and the targets set in the Plan could well raise expectations about what the NHS can deliver, thereby risking greater disappointment if it fails to do so.

Soon the responsibility for spending the NHS budget will pass entirely to primary care trusts (PCTs). The Department of Health states that it will give PCTs greater freedom to spend more of the money as they see fit. But central priorities will remain in place, as will many of the financial pressures described above. It remains to be seen whether they will be better able to balance the books, as well as squeezing more out of the system to deliver the improvements that the Government is hoping for.

1 Health Authority Revenue Resource Limits Exposition Book. *http://www.doh. gov.uk/allocations/2001-2002/#expo* (viewed 18 July 2001).

2 Secretary of State for Health. *The NHS Plan: a plan for investment; a plan for reform.* Cm 4818-I. London: Stationery Office, 2000. *http://www.doh.gov.uk/nhsplan/default.htm*

3 Health Authority Revenue Resource Limits Exposition Book. *Op. cit.*

4 Department of Health. *The Government expenditure plans 2001–2002 to 2003–2004 and main estimates.* Cm 5103. London: Stationery Office, 2001. *http://www.doh.gov. uk/dohreport/report2001/drforwa/pdf* (viewed 18 July 2001).

5 Ford J. The BMA funding review. In: Appleby J, Harrison A. *Health care UK. Spring 2001.* London: King's Fund, 2001.

6 Department of Health. *NHS Plan implementation programme.* London: Department of Health, 2001. *http://www. doh.gov.uk.nhsplanimpprogramme/index.htm* (viewed 18 July 2001).

7 *Ibid.*

8 Report of the Controller and Auditor General. *NHS (England) summarised accounts 1999–2000.* London: National Audit Office, 12 July 2001. *http://www. nao.gov.uk/pn/01-02/0102119.htm* (viewed 18 July 2001).

Key events in health care

Anthony Harrison

OVERVIEW

The return to power of Labour at the beginning of June has meant that the agenda for the months covered in this review calendar was largely set by earlier events, of which the publication of the NHS Plan was clearly the most important. The calendar records a number of announcements bearing on priority areas – cancer, mental health and heart disease – and also on the recruitment of the extra staff needed to implement the Plan's proposals.

Although the Plan has set the general direction of the Government's policy towards the NHS, there have been some surprises; in particular, the proposals for the reform of the structure of the NHS contained in *Shifting the Balance of Power within the NHS* (on 7 September). This proposes a radical shift in the structure of the NHS – most significantly the abolition of health authorities and their replacement by a much smaller number of strategic authorities. It also appears to suggest that the Government intends to decentralise the NHS by giving more

power to the 'frontline' by, for example, handing over 75 per cent of the health budget to primary care trusts. At the same time, however, it has shown no enthusiasm for abandoning the range of targets that hospitals and others must meet. Whether localities will gain a significant degree of discretion over the funds at their disposal remains unclear.

The Plan was criticised at the time of its publication for giving too much emphasis to service development to the neglect of preventive measures and the wider public health agenda. In August, the Government responded by publishing its plans for developing the public health role (9 August) and for tackling health inequalities (23 August).

This calendar also reports some other very important developments, of which perhaps the most significant is the publication of the report of the Bristol Inquiry (18 July). The report makes a large number of sweeping proposals for the reform of how the NHS operates, emphasising in particular the need for the culture of the Service to change if it is genuinely to focus on the patient. The Government responded quickly with a small number of announcements, e.g. of the unification of professional regulation (9 August), which were already in the pipeline. A more detailed response to the report is to be made in the autumn. In September, however, there were two announcements bearing on the role of patients within the NHS. On 3 September, the Government put forward its revised proposals for patient representation on NHS bodies and on 14 September plans for the development of the expert patient role were published.

JUNE

25 **Personal medical services:** fourth wave of personal medical service pilots announced. They are intended to:

- have a clear focus on public health
- offer new approaches to addressing the needs of deprived areas/ vulnerable groups tackling inequalities in health
- tackle recruitment issues in under-doctored areas
- propose closer working with social care
- promote access
- be whole PCG/T pilots
- be PMS Plus pilots, providing a range of extended services
- utilise GPs with a specialist interest
- indicate innovative use of primary health care team roles.

27 **Quality of care:** joint statement issued by Government and medical profession on quality of care. The statement contains a seven-point pledge that the Government, the medical profession and the NHS have signed up to:

- to continue to show a commitment from the top to implementing the programme of quality assurance and quality improvement
- to take every opportunity to involve patients and their representatives in decisions about their own care and in the planning and design of services
- to work towards providing valid, reliable, up-to-date information on the quality of health services
- to work together in determining clinical priorities
- to create a culture within the NHS which is open and participative, where learning and evaluation are prominent, and which recognises safety and the needs of patients as paramount
- to recognise that in a service as large and complex as the NHS things will sometimes go wrong. Without lessening commitment to safety and public accountability of services, to recognise that honest failure should not be responded to primarily by blame and retribution, but by learning and by a drive to reduce risk for future patients
- to recognise that the professions, the Government and the public share a common interest and commitment to improving the quality of services for patients. Minor disagreements on points of detail must not be allowed to obscure this common goal (PR 2001/0284).

28 **NHS Direct:** project announced in the West Midlands which allows about 50,000 digital TV users to book appointments with their GP, get general and local health information and to speak to NHS Direct nurses on screen.

29 **Ambulance services:** £10 million of Lottery money allocated by the New Opportunities Fund to improve ambulance services.

JULY

4 **Prostate cancer:** Government announces that a series or measures is to be taken to ensure that men get more information about the risks of prostate cancer. A web site is to be launched consisting of patient experiences: www.dipex.org

5 **Heart disease:** Government announces that £110 million of Lottery money will be targeted at areas with the highest rates of heart disease. The money is to be spent on more up-to-date equipment and for specialist laboratories for diagnosis, and to improve cardiac rehabilitation.

6 **GP contract:** NHS Confederation asked to take forward negotiations for a new GP contract.

9 **Mental health:** establishment of the National Mental Health Institute in England announced. Its first task is to develop a national research plan and to set up a network of leading institutions to work collaboratively. This will be responsible for the creation of a research infrastructure to run large clinical trials. It is intended to:

- require the contributions of all parties including but not exclusively: health, social care, the non-statutory sector and the service user and carer movements
- guide consistent implementation of what is the most radical reform of mental health services ever

- ensure best practice and best evidence gets into common practice
- be underpinned by a sound set of principles and values
- be driven by the needs of service users, their families, friends and communities
- set Mental Health Service development in the wider context of community development, regeneration and social inclusion.

10 **Compensation:** committee established under Chief Medical Officer Liam Donaldson to improve the existing system for clinical negligence compensation. Its remit will include exploration of the following:

- no fault compensation – which may save time and costs in achieving settlements. This system would encourage a more open system by not blaming staff
- structured settlements – instead of a lump sum, patients would receive periodic payments based on their future needs, including nursing care or other treatment
- fixed tariff schemes for specific injuries
- mediation – greater use of mediation for resolving disputes.

12 **NHS structure:** proposals published for the reform of the structure of the NHS and the Department of Health. *Shifting the Balance of Power within the NHS* proposes that primary care trusts become the lead organisations for assessing needs, planning and securing all health services and improving health. Existing health authorities to be replaced by 30 Strategic Health Authorities

(StHAs), and within NHS trusts greater responsibilities are to be delegated to clinical teams and networks.

Within the Department of Health, the changes are intended to lead to:

- a smaller number of priorities
- a single top team working across health and social care
- an open approach to involving stakeholders and partners
- a determination to decentralise activity and authority
- a focus on doing only those things that only it can.

13 **Staffing:** Government announces that since April 2001 nearly 3000 nurses and midwives returned to the NHS or have been training to return.

16 **Flu immunisation:** target set of minimum 65 per cent uptake in those aged 65 and over. The aim is also to improve uptake among those most at risk in younger age groups, including those with the following conditions:

- chronic respiratory disease, including asthma
- chronic heart disease
- chronic renal disease
- diabetes
- immunosuppression.

18 **Bristol Inquiry:** following publication of the Inquiry report, the Government announced that a national director of children's healthcare services would be appointed, a new Office for Information on Healthcare Performance would be set up within the Commission for Health Improvement, and a new overarching

council for regulating health care professions would be established (see entry below).

23 **Cancer care:** national project launched to cut waiting times for patients with stomach cancer. A total of £2.5 million is being made available to provide more training opportunities for staff in endoscopy.

23 **Drugs:** 26 pilot schemes announced with the National Medicines Management programme.

Generics: discussion paper published, setting out options for the reform of the supply of generic drugs.

Antibiotic resistance: new advisory committee announced, in response to House of Lords report on resistance to antibiotics.

25 **Cancer care:** £2 million allocated to educate and support community nurses in providing care to cancer patients at home.

NHS Plus: trusts asked to propose their occupational services for membership of NHS Plus.

26 **Smoking:** Government announces that the NHS has helped 61,000 people to give up smoking in the previous year.

27 **Sexual health:** the first national strategy of sexual health and HIV services launched. Key elements of the strategy include:

- the first ever national information campaign aimed at the general public, to span prevention of sexually transmitted infections,

HIV and unintended pregnancy, to safeguard sexual health

- new targets to reduce the number of newly acquired HIV infections and gonorrhoea infections
- targeted screening for chlamydia to be phased in from next year
- a model for sexual health services that can be delivered by every PCT, increasing access and bringing a broader role for nurses and other staff working in primary care
- routine HIV testing to be offered in all sexual health clinics to reduce the number of undiagnosed cases
- more people to be offered hepatitis B vaccine in sexual health clinics to protect them against sexually transmitted infection
- new one-stop sexual health services to be piloted and evaluated
- local stakeholders will review sexual health and HIV services in each area and ensure that sexual health services are delivered in each PCT (PR 2001/0354).

31 **Ward improvement:** ward sisters allowed to apply for charge cards to enable them to spend up to £5000 on ward improvements.

AUGUST

2 **Children's services:** standards for children receiving care in hospitals to be set as first steps towards a National Service Framework for Children.

8 **Smoking:** campaign launched to reduced to the level of smoking and tobacco chewing in Asian communities.

Hospitals: NHS buys The Heart Hospital from Gleneagles Hospital UK.

9 **Regulation:** the Council for the Regulation of Healthcare announced. It will oversee the work of all the existing regulatory bodies. The Council should:

- explicitly puts patients' interests first
- be open and transparent, and allow for robust public scrutiny
- ensure that the existing regulatory bodies act in a more consistent manner
- provide for greater integration and co-ordination between the regulatory bodies and the sharing of good practice and information
- require the regulatory bodies to conform to principles of good regulation
- promote continuous improvement through the setting of new performance targets and monitoring (PR 2001/0374).

Public health: *From Vision to Reality* published, which records the action being taken in the public health field.

Nurse prescribing: consultation launched on the scope of the prescribing of prescription-only medicines by nurses to enable them to treat or provide:

- minor ailments, such as hay fever and acne
- minor injuries, such as burns, cuts and sprains
- health promotion and maintenance, such as providing vitamins for women who are planning pregnancy
- palliative care.

22 **Service reconfiguration:** Dr Peter Barret appointed head of the Independent Reconfiguration Panel. This will assess proposed changes against clear criteria, such as:

- quality of care
- community health needs
- accessibility
- patient safety
- clinical and service quality (PR 2001/0388).

Medicines: proposals for clearer labelling of medicines announced by Committee on Safety of Medicines. The Committee recommends:

- A standard format for the labelling of all medicines. The new 'number plate' will clearly identify and carry details of the safe use of the medicine. This will allow both health professionals and patients to check at a glance that a) the medicine prescribed is the correct one; and b) how it should be administered or taken.
- The redesign of labels and packaging, for example, using colour and design to make medicines more individually identifiable. This will give patients more confidence when self-medicating and will help to ensure that they take their medicines as prescribed.
- That other strategies could be used for specific medicines to support labelling improvements, for example, co-ordinating the colour of the tablets themselves with the colour of the packaging, making them more individually identifiable. This will help both health professionals and patients to easily distinguish between the

medicines they administer or take, helping to reduce cases of medication error.
- That all new labelling will be user tested by the drugs companies to ensure that it is clear and understandable to all patients, and that commercial information on labelling does not impinge on patient information or weaken its clarity (PR 2001/0387).

23 **Health inequalities:** consultation paper launched. It sets out the following priority areas:

- providing a sure foundation through healthy pregnancy and early childhood
- improving opportunity for children and young people
- improving NHS primary care services
- tackling the major killers – coronary heart disease and cancer
- strengthening disadvantaged communities
- tackling the wider determinants of health inequalities (PR 2001/0389).

29 **Clinical negligence:** discussion document, *Call for Ideas*, published, seeking views on how to reform the current arrangements.

Cleft lip and palate services: guidance issued to the NHS on appointments to cleft lip and palate services, following the report from the Clinical Services Advisory Committee.

30 **Dental health:** one million children to receive free toothbrushes and toothpaste over three years. The programme will be targeted on areas

in London, the north-west and Yorkshire, where dental decay is at a particularly high level.

SEPTEMBER

3   **Public involvement:** proposals launched to give patients and the public a greater say in the running of the NHS:

- a new national body called 'Voice – the Commission for Patient and Public Involvement in Health'
- Patients' Forums for every NHS trust and PCT to inspect NHS services, including casualty watch checks, and ensure that patients' concerns are dealt with rapidly and to everyone's satisfaction
- local bodies, to be called 'Voice', that will report patients' concerns from PALs and forums to the new Strategic Health Authorities (StHAs) and facilitate public involvement in the NHS (PR 2001/0401).

6   **Recruitment:** Starter Home Initiative announced to assist NHS staff to buy housing in parts of London and the South.

7   **NHS structure:** consultation proposals published for new health authority boundaries. The document proposes that:

- by 2002, two-thirds of existing health authorities will have disappeared as they merge
- the 30 or so that remain will become Strategic Health Authorities (StHAs), each covering an average population of 1.5 million
- the new boundaries for the StHAs

will broadly correspond to clinical networks, such as those for cancer services, and line up alongside local authority and Government Office boundaries (PR 2001/0413).

10 **Staffing:** plans announced for the creation of 124 nurse, midwife and health visitor consultant staff.

11 **Staffing:** recruitment drive launched to raise the number of allied health professionals including health care scientists working in the NHS.

14 **Patients:** *The Expert Patient: A New Approach to Chronic Disease Management* published. Following the recommendations of the report:

- User led groups will be set up in local NHS services to enable people living with long-term medical conditions to share their knowledge and skills to help others to better manage their conditions. Pilot groups will be set up by all PCTs between 2001 and 2004, and following an extensive evaluation the programme will be rolled out across the NHS between 2004 and 2007.
- A core course will be established to promote health professionals' knowledge and understanding about the benefits – for them as well as the patients – of user-led self-management programmes.
- A National Co-ordinating and Training Resource Centre will be set up to provide training and current information to help health, social services and voluntary sector professionals keep up to date with developments in the provision of self-management.

Kidney services: membership announced of the external reference group for the Renal National Service Framework. This is to be published in four modules:

- effective delivery of dialysis
- transplantation
- primary prevention and pre-dialysis
- alternative models of care.

20 **Medical devices:** Lord Hunt identifies areas of concern in the regulation of medical devices:

- the need to reclassify some higher risk devices so they will be subjected to stricter controls
- manufacturers not always having accurate and relevant clinical data on the performance of their devices
- variations in the standards and performance of the independent certification bodies – known as Certified Bodies – that check that devices comply with EU Regulations (PR 2001/0434).

21 **Heart and lung transplants:** consultation document issued proposing new national standards for heart and lung services, covering:

- staffing levels and qualifications
- arrangements for retrieval of organs
- the number of transplants carried out or number of patients seen in follow-up clinics
- survival and rejection rates.

Hospitals: the formation of the Better Hospital Food Panel announced. This will advise on the future direction of the Better Hospital Food Programme and identify new standards for food services in the NHS.

25 **Hospitals:** the first performance tables for hospitals published. The best performing trusts are to be granted ten key freedoms:

- less frequent monitoring from the centre
- fewer and better co-ordinated inspections
- development of their own investment programmes without receiving prior approval
- retention of more of the proceeds of local land sales for re-investment in local services
- becoming pilot sites for new initiatives, such as team bonuses for staff
- extra cash for central programmes without having to bid for it
- extra resources if they are required to take over and improve the performance of persistently failing trusts
- the ability to create new 'spin-out' companies to extend their research strengths, or sell services to other organisations. Profits from these ventures will be reinvested in patient care
- the opportunity for chief executives to provide direct advice and input to ministers and the NHS Chief Executive in the preparation of new national policies and the review of existing ones
- the opportunity for chief executives to join the learning set, which will consider additional freedoms for their organisations and an early involvement in the succession planning and development programme being constructed by NHS Chief Executive Nigel Crisp (PR 2001/0440).

APPENDIX

NHS Plan targets

John Appleby

A plan would not be a plan without targets, and implementation documents supporting the NHS Plan (see, for example, *http://www.doh.gov.uk/nhsplanimpprogramme/index. htm*) provide details of the main targets and milestones the NHS has been set.

ACCESS: Waiting times, booked admissions, NHS Direct, cancelled operations

SERVICE AREA	TARGET	BY...
Inpatients	Reduce the number of over-12-month waits and implement a maximum waiting time of 15 months	March 2002
Inpatients	Reduce maximum wait for inpatient treatment to six months	2005
Outpatients	Reduce the number of over-13-week waits and implement a maximum waiting time of 26 weeks	March 2002
Outpatients	Reduce the maximum wait for an outpatients appointment to three months	2005
Outpatient outreach	All PCG/Ts to have agreed with their main providers plans to deliver outpatient consultations in primary/community settings	2002
Cancer: waiting	Maximum one-month wait from urgent GP referral to treatment for testicular cancer, children's cancers and leukaemia	December 2001

ACCESS: continued

SERVICE AREA	TARGET	BY...
Cancer: waiting	Maximum one-month wait from diagnosis to treatment for breast cancer	December 2001
Cancer: waiting	Maintain maximum two-week wait for first outpatient appointment for patients referred urgently with suspected cancers	ongoing
Waiting lists	Maintain the commitment to cut waiting lists by 100,000 from the 1997 level	ongoing
A&E	75% of patients attending A&E to wait four hours or less from arrival to admission, transfer or discharge	March 2002
A&E	100% of patients admitted to hospital via A&E to be found a bed within four hours of a decision to admit	March 2002
Booked admissions	Every acute trust to be booking at least two specialties or high-volume procedures	March 2001
Booked admissions	5 million patients will have benefited from the Booked Admissions Programme	March 2002
Booked admissions	Two-thirds of all outpatient appointments and inpatient elective admissions will be pre-booked	2003/04
Booked admissions	100% of all outpatient appointments and inpatient elective admissions will be pre-booked	2005
Operations	Patients whose operation are cancelled by a hospital on the day of surgery for non-clinical reasons will be offered another binding date within a maximum of the next 28 days or have their treatment at the time and hospital of the patient's choice	March 2002
NHS Direct	Everyone will be able to see an NHS dentist by phoning NHS Direct	September 2001

ACCESS: continued

SERVICE AREA	TARGET	BY...
NHS Direct	NHS Direct to refer people, where appropriate, to help from their local pharmacy	December 2002
General practice	60% of patients to wait no more than 24 hours for an appointment with a primary health care professional and no more than 48 hours for an appointment with a GP	March 2002
General practice	All health authorities to have commissioned Occupational Health Services for all GPs and their staff	April 2002
One-stop centres	500 one-stop centres will have been established, bringing primary and community services – and where possible social services – together under one roof	2004

QUALITY

SERVICE AREA	TARGET	BY...
Adverse health care events	All NHS organisations to have local systems in place to report to the new national full mandatory reporting scheme for adverse health care events (as in *An Organisation with a Memory*)	January 2002
Patient consent	Changes to ensure good consent practice introduced throughout the NHS	2001
Hospital food	All hospitals to provide a 24-hour food service to patients, which reflects the new NHS national menu to be launched in April 2001, and which meets or exceeds the standards set. All hospitals to have quality monitoring arrangements that take account of patient views and which ensure that food meets patient need in terms of quality, presentation and quantity, and is genuinely available at all times of day and night	December 2001
Mixed-sex wards	95% of mixed-sex accommodation has been eliminated	December 2002

QUALITY: continued

SERVICE AREA	TARGET	BY...
Ward nurse-held budgets	All hospitals to have in place senior sisters and charge nurses, easily accessible by patients, who must be given the necessary resources to sort out the fundamentals of care, in the form of a ward environment budget, which every trust and PCT, where appropriate, is required to provide. Each budget will be worth a minimum of £5000 in 2001/02	April 2002
Hospital cleanliness	All hospitals to invest to meet standards of cleanliness set out in their Cleanliness Action Plan and to routinely monitor patients' views on the cleanliness of hospitals	April 2001
Ward housekeepers	Introduce ward housekeepers	December 2004

PATIENTS' VIEWS

SERVICE AREA	TARGET	BY...
Patient & carer views	All NHS organisations, as well as care homes, to be monitoring patient and carer experience and satisfaction on a rigorous, comparable and systematic basis and publish in a Patient Prospectus the views received and action taken as a result, in accordance with forthcoming guidance	March 2002
Patient forums	All NHS trusts and primary care trusts to have Patient Advocacy & Liaison Service and Patient Forums in line with forthcoming guidance, and all health authorities to have established Independent Local Advisory Forums	April 2002
Patient's Charter replacement	All parts of the NHS to be implementing the NHS Plan standards contained within *Your guide to the NHS*, which will replace the current *Patient's Charter*	April 2001

PATIENTS' VIEW: continued

SERVICE AREA	TARGET	BY...
Patient communication	All NHS trusts will have made progress towards letters between clinicians about an individual patient's care being copied to the patient as of right	April 2002

CANCER SERVICES:

SERVICE AREA	TARGET	BY...
Deaths	Reduce the mortality rates from cancer by at least 20% in people under 75 years of age	2010
Drugs	Ensure all patients receive the clinically proven and cost-effective drugs they need, taking full account of NICE appraisals of 13 chemotherapy treatments to be published in summer 2001	2001
Improving Outcomes Guidance	Improve quality of treatment patients receive by beginning to implement the Improving Outcomes Guidance on gynaecological, upper gastrointestinal, urological and haematological cancers	no date
Smoking Help	50,000 smokers quit, four weeks after starting smoking cessation intervention, with particular emphasis on manual socio-economic groups	March 2002
Smoking	Deliver a decrease of at least 1% in the proportion of pregnant women who continue to smoke during pregnancy	2001/02
Palliative care	All cancer networks to develop costed strategic plans for palliative care in partnership with voluntary organisations, to begin implementation in 2001	2001

CANCER SERVICES: continued

SERVICE AREA	TARGET	BY...
Cancer networks	Cancer networks to develop and begin implementing strategic service delivery plans to cover all aspects of cancer services including workforce, education and training requirements	2001
Equipment	All Regions to develop cancer facilities strategies for equipment to keep the stock of equipment up to date and to work towards a fair distribution of equipment. The regional strategies must ensure in aggregate that their plans make sufficient progress towards the NHS	ongoing
Equipment	50 new MRI cancer scanners, 200 new CT cancer scanners, 80 new liquid cytology units and 45 new linear accelerators	2004
Fruit & vegetables	Each health authority to prepare quantified plans to increase access to and consumption of vegetables and fruit, particularly among those on low incomes, to support the national five-a-day programme	2001
Inequalities	Health communities must demonstrate in their plans that the essential requirements of the NHS Cancer Plan will be delivered, with particular emphasis on tackling inequalities and improving health	ongoing

HEART DISEASE

SERVICE AREA	TARGET	BY...
Deaths	Reduce substantially the mortality rates from heart disease by at least 40% in people aged under 75	2010
Revascularisations	The national target is to achieve, ahead of time, the original target of 3000 additional procedures over the 1999/2000 baseline and make progress towards bringing on-stream at least an extra 3000 on top of this	2003

HEART DISEASE: continued

SERVICE AREA	TARGET	BY...
Ambulance calls	Deliver and maintain the standard of 75% of category 'A' ambulance calls receiving a first response within eight minutes	2001/02
Thrombolysis	75% of eligible patients to receive thrombolysis within 30 minutes of hospital arrival	March 2002
Effective prescribing	More than 80% of people discharged from hospital following a heart attack will be prescribed clinically and cost-effective medicines (especially aspirin, beta-blockers and statins)	March 2002
Primary care records	Every practice should have all medical records and hospital correspondence held in a way that allows them to be retrieved readily in date order	no date
Primary care records	Every practice should have appropriate medical records containing easily discernible drug therapy lists for patients on long-term therapy	no date
Primary care	Practices should use their systems to deliver structured care, including appropriate drug therapies to people with CHD	no date
Equipment	Health communities should take full advantage of the CHD NSF and NHS Plan pledge to invest in a wide range of equipment and facilities to support achievement of these targets, including a further 3000 automated defibrillators, which will be made available in public places	no date
Training & education	Health communities should develop costed workforce plans, including education and training, to support implementation of the NSF	no date

MENTAL HEALTH

SERVICE AREA	TARGET	BY...
Deaths	Reduce substantially the mortality rates from suicide and undetermined injury by at least 20%	2010
National Service Framework	Local Implementation Teams to be signed off by the relevant NHS and Social Care Regional Office, their Stage 3 plan for implementing the mental health NSF, and the mental health targets in the NHS Plan	November 2001
Assertive outreach	Every health authority to identify all clients who require the assertive outreach approach, and prepare plans for a further 50 assertive outreach teams to ensure that all clients who need this approach will be in receipt of such services by 2003	March 2002
Re-admissions	National psychiatric re-admission rate must be reduced to 12.3%	March 2002
Specialist mental health service users	All specialist mental health service users on enhanced CPA should have a written care plan, available on an electronic information system at all trust operational bases	March 2001
Primary/specialist care links	All health authorities should have in place protocols agreed and implemented between primary care and specialist mental health services for the management of: depression and postnatal depression; anxiety disorders; schizophrenia; those requiring psychological therapies; and drug and alcohol dependence	March 2001
Patient information	Health authorities need to ensure that information about treatment and services are available for all people presenting in primary care with mental health problems, including information about access to local self-help groups and support services such as housing and employment	March 2002

MENTAL HEALTH: continued

SERVICE AREA	TARGET	BY...
Suicide prevention	To help prevent suicides among high-risk groups, by all patients with a current or recent history of severe mental illness and/or deliberate self-harm, and in particular those who at some time during their admission were detained under the Mental Health Act because of a high risk of suicide, must be followed up by a face-to-face contact with a mental health professional within seven days of discharge from inpatient hospital care. Also, every health authority and local council to have multi-agency protocols agreed and operational for the sharing of information relevant to reducing risk of serious harm to self or others	March 2002
Prison services	60 staff will be recruited to provide prison in-reach services at selected prisons and 40 new secure beds will be provided to transfer those people no longer requiring the conditions of high security	March 2002

OLDER PEOPLE

SERVICE AREA	TARGET	BY...
Avoidable hospitalisation	At least 130,000 people to benefit from reductions in preventable hospitalisation and year-on-year reductions in delays in moving people aged 75 and over on from hospital	no date
National Service Framework	National Service Framework for Older People to be implemented	from April 2001
Health/social care assessment	Introduce a single assessment process for health and social care, including a proactive process to identify and invite more vulnerable people for assessment	April 2002
Delayed transfers	Average rate of delayed transfer of care for people 75 and over to be 10%, approximately equating to a reduction of 1000 beds occupied by people aged 75 and over awaiting transfer of care in comparison to 2000/01 level	during 2001/02

OLDER PEOPLE: continued

SERVICE AREA	TARGET	BY...
Emergency admissions	Average growth in the per capita rate of emergency admissions for people aged 75 and over to be less than 2%	2001/02
Emergency re-admissions	The rate of emergency re-admissions within 28 days of discharge to stay the same or decrease	2001/02
Intermediate care	1500 more intermediate care beds	2001/02
Intermediate care	60,000 more people to receive intermediate care services	2001/02
Equipment services	Develop and start to implement plans for integrating community equipment services and for increasing the number of service users	2001/02
Respite care	25,000 more carers to benefit from respite/breaks services	2001/02
Independence	The number of older people helped to live at home per 1000 of the population aged 65 or over to increase by at least 2% nationally	2001/02
Flu vaccine	Increase the uptake of flu vaccine for winter 2001/02	2001/02
Nursing homes	NHS to be ready to assume responsibility for arranging and funding registered nursing care for people in nursing homes. Joint assessment procedures with social care will need to take account of this realigned responsibility for everyone whose care needs are assessed or reviewed	October 2001
Private sector	Every health authority and local council to work with its local independent sector providers to determine what nursing and residential beds are needed in the future subject to securing the right levels of quality and value for money	ongoing

CHILDREN

SERVICE AREA	TARGET	BY...
Health inequalities	National health inequalities targets to be developed	early 2001
Health inequalities	National health poverty index to be developed	2002
Disabled children	6000 extra severely disabled children to receive support services	April 2002
CAMHS Development Strategy	All health authorities and local councils to have an agreed joint CAMHS Development Strategy that sets out how local and national priorities are to be met, including 24-hour cover and outreach services, and increasing early intervention and prevention programmes for children	May 2001
CAMHS beds	Provide an extra 30 CAMHS in-patient beds	March 2002
Health and antenatal screening	Health authorities, with other relevant agencies, to prepare for the co-ordination, extension and quality improvement of children's health and antenatal screening programmes by putting in place an infrastructure for delivering change effectively	March 2002
Teenage pregnancy	Health authorities and local councils to produce a joint report demonstrating satisfactory progress in implementing their agreed ten-year teenage pregnancy strategy	March 2002
Teenage pregnancy	Demonstrate progress towards agreed local targets of a 15% reduction in under-18 conception rates	2004
Teenage pregnancy	Reduction in under-18 conception rates in the range of 40–60%	2010
Youth Offending Teams	Contribute fully to every Youth Offending Team, including undertaking a review of the resources, both staffing and revenue, required by YOTs from health and social services to properly assess the needs of children and young people at risk of offending and to develop a service programme accordingly	

CHILDREN: continued

SERVICE AREA	TARGET	BY...
Sure Start	Contribute fully to any local Sure Start programmes and to develop 250 such programmes	2002
General practice	Increase the number of GPs in deprived areas. By then a third of all GPs will be working in PMS and it is expected that a majority of these PMS pilots will be working in deprived communities	2002
Education	Improve the level of education, training and employment outcomes for care leavers aged 19, so that levels for this group are at least 75% of those achieved by all young people in the same area	March 2004
Education	Increase the percentage of children in care who achieve at least five GCSEs at grade A*–C to 15%	2004
Adoption	Maximise the contribution adoption can make to providing permanent families for children	no date
Adoption	Develop and improve post-adoption support services, including health services provided to adoptive families, to increase successful adoptive placements	no date
Adoption	11 specified councils will work with the Adoption and Permanence Taskforce to improve performance and spread best practice	from December 2000
Looked after children	Give children the care and guidance needed to narrow the gap between the proportion of children in care and their peers who have been given a final warning or have been convicted	2004

CHILDREN: continued

SERVICE AREA	TARGET	BY...
Looked after children	All councils to complete a rapid scrutiny of the number of looked after children waiting for adoption for more than six months and approved adopters who have been waiting for more than six months to be matched with an appropriate child. Identify where avoidable delays are occurring and take steps to rectify the position	January 2001
Looked after children	No more than 16% of children in care should have three or more placements in any council	March 2001
Looked after children	Every looked-after child to have an annual health assessment and a personal education plan	no date
Looked after children	Demonstrate that the level of employment, training or education among young people aged 19 in 2001/02 who were looked after by councils in their 17th year on 1 April 1999 is at least 60% of the level among all young people of the same age in the same area	2001/02
Looked after children	12,000 young people to receive help under the new leaving care arrangements	April 2002
Education	Increase to at least 50% the proportion of children leaving care at 16 or later with a GCSE or GNVQ qualification	March 2001
Education	Increase to at least 75% the proportion of children leaving care at 16 or later with a GCSE or GNVQ qualification	2003

DRUG MISUSE

SERVICE AREA	TARGET	BY...
Treatment programmes	Increase the participation of problem drug users in drug treatment programmes by 55%	2004
Treatment programmes	Increase the participation of problem drug users in drug treatment programmes by 100%	2008
Treatment programmes	15% more problem drug misusers per health authority (excluding criminal justice clients), and 10% more per local authority accessing drug treatment services	March 2002
Waiting times	All Drug Action Teams to set maximum waiting times for each type of treatment to achieve the performance of the top 25%	March 2002

EFFICIENCY

SERVICE AREA	TARGET	BY...
Benchmark target	The level of efficiency achieved by trusts providing the best care across the country (as defined by the Performance Assessment Framework domains of access, outcomes and effectiveness) to provide the benchmark for the rest of the NHS	2005
Best Value	Each NHS organisation to review at least one major service each year in line with the 'Best Value' regime	begin in 2001/02
Earned autonomy	All NHS bodies will be expected to make progress towards a position of earned autonomy, making year-on-year improvements in overall levels of performance, measured by the achievement of a 'green light' status for performance	no date
Earned autonomy	PCGs and PCTs to consider extending the earned autonomy approach to their member practices and other PMS providers through appropriate use of indicative budgets, incentives and clinical governance	no date

BEDS & EQUIPMENT

SERVICE AREA	TARGET	BY...
National Bed Inquiry	Health authorities, NHS trusts and PCG/Ts will be expected to audit themselves against the National Beds Inquiry templates. Such an audit will help health authorities to assess their future requirements for beds in line with the findings of the NBI and the requirements set out in the NHS Plan	no date
Beds	7000 extra NHS beds, of which 2100 will be general and acute beds	2004
Beds	5000 extra intermediate care beds	2004
Beds	30% increase in adult critical care beds over next 3 years	2004
New capital schemes	Regional Offices to ensure that, in aggregate, new capital schemes (including Private Finance Initiative) lead to an overall increase in the number of general and acute beds	
Equipment	50 new MRI cancer scanners	2004
Equipment	200 new CT cancer scanners	2004
Equipment	80 new liquid cytology units	2004
Equipment	45 new linear accelerators	2004
GP premises	Up to 3000 family doctors' premises will be substantially refurbished or replaced	2004

STAFF

SERVICE AREA	TARGET	BY...
Staff involvement	NHS organisations to establish action plans for increasing staff involvement in planning and decision-making	no date
Consultants	7500 more consultants	2004

STAFF: continued

SERVICE AREA	TARGET	BY...
GPs	At least 2000 more GPs	2004
Nurses	20,000 extra nurses	2004
Therapists	6500 extra therapists	2004
Training places	Through the postgraduate deaneries, it is expected that increases of at least 300 specialist registrar and 150 GP registrar numbers will be delivered	2001/02
Training places	Workforce Development Confederations working with their local health communities will be expected to deliver an increase of 1 000 nurse training commissions and at least 700 PAMs training commissions	no date
Nurse consultants	The creation of more nurse, midwife and health visitor consultant posts	during 2001/02
Nurse consultants	The introduction of therapist consultants	during 2001/02
Key roles for nurses	Full implementation of the Chief Nursing Officer's 'Ten Key Roles for Nurses'	during 2001/02
Nurse prescribing	The majority of nurses to be able to supply or prescribe medicines	2004
Continuing professional development	Explicit local action, with accountability at board level, to co-ordinate and deliver continuing professional development for all professional groups linked to strategic initiatives at confederation and regional office level	no date
Staff accommodation	Increases staff accommodation by 1500 new units	April 2002
Child care	Improved child care provision, including 20 new nurseries	April 2002

STAFF: continued

SERVICE AREA	TARGET	BY...
Individual Learning Accounts	Health communities to have schemes in place to guarantee that a third of all eligible staff will have access to either vocational training or Individual Learning Accounts	March 2002
Personal development plans	In line with the Working Together target, the majority of health professional staff should have personal development plans. Personal development planning should be extended to all staff groups with particular emphasis on work-and team-based learning and development planning	no date
Student support scheme	Social services to review their arrangements for recruiting and retaining staff and ensuring staff are adequately trained so that the right staff and in the right numbers are available to deliver quality services. From 2001/02, £41 million over three years will be made available to local councils specifically for the establishment of a student support scheme for those studying for first level professional social work qualifications	no date

INFORMATION SYSTEMS

SERVICE AREA	TARGET	BY...
GP networks	100% of GPs connected to NHSnet	March 2002
Network access	Connecting users: all NHS staff to have basic common desktop and NHSnet connection	March 2003
Electronic book-in	Delivering integrated services: all bookings for patient care to be made electronically	March 2005
Electronic records	Electronic records: all NHS organisations to have EPRs and EHRs in place to deliver effective services	March 2005

INFORMATION SYSTEMS: continued

SERVICE AREA	TARGET	BY...
Electronic records	Local councils will need to take forward the action identified in the consultation paper *Information for Social Care*. Best practice will be identified in order to take forward the concept of an electronic social care record related to the electronic health record	no date
Computer users	All desktop users to have full NHS Address Book	March 2002
Computer users	All desktop users to have NHS Number Tracing	March 2003
Computer users	All desktop users to have NHS Payroll and HR	March 2004

Statistical trends (and NHS Plan targets)

John Appleby

WAITING LIST/TIMES

Inpatients and day cases waiting >6 months

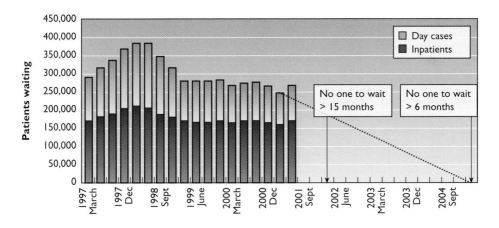

GP referrals waiting over 13 weeks to be seen in outpatients

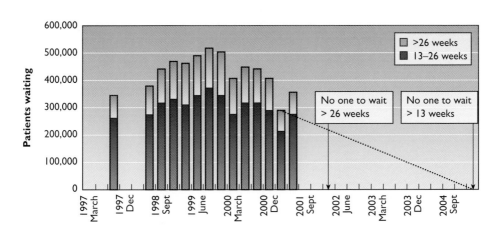

Numbers of suspected breast cancer patients waiting over two weeks for outpatient appointments following an urgent referral within 24 hours of GP decision to refer

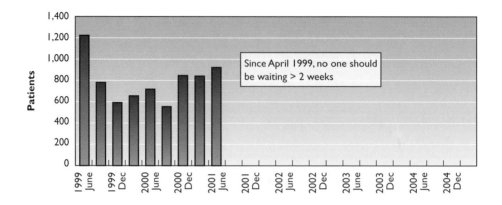

Total waiting lists

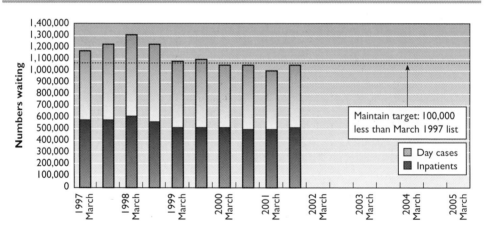

Mean and median waiting times: inpatients and day cases

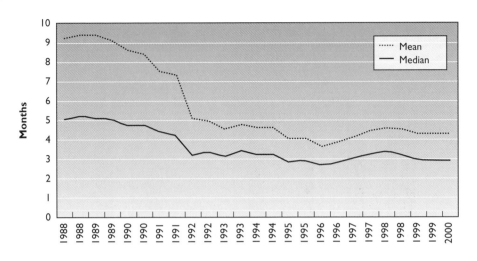

PUBLIC ATTITUDES

Dissatisfaction with the NHS: percentage stating very or quite dissatisfied

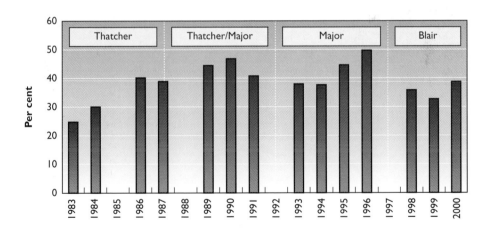

Dissatisfaction with hospital care: percentage stating very or quite dissatisfied

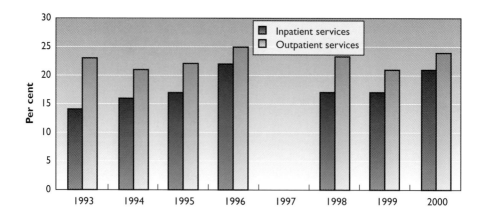

Dissatisfaction with GPs and dentists: percentage stating very or quite dissatisfied

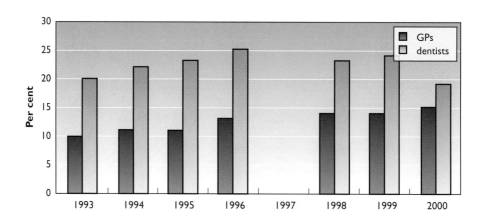

Percentage who say the following in need of a lot or some improvement

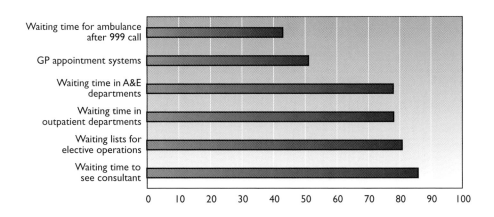

FUNDING

Percentage change in UK NHS net real spending (deflated by HCHS specific inflation)

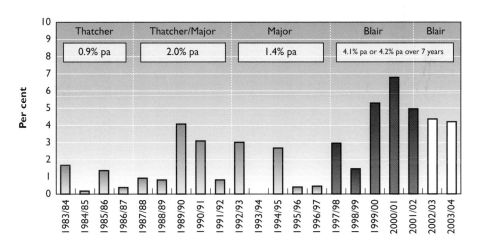

UK NHS spending as a percentage of GDP

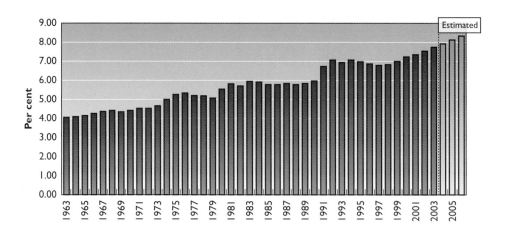

BEDS

Acute bed availability: England

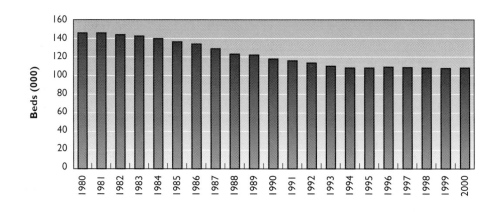

ACTIVITY

Percentage change in numbers of inpatients and day cases

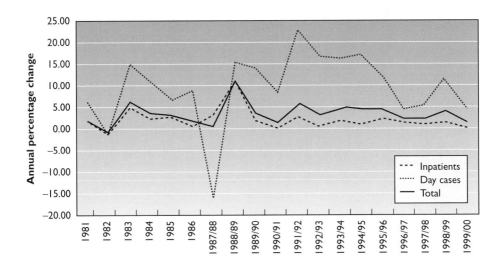

Ordinary and day case activity: England

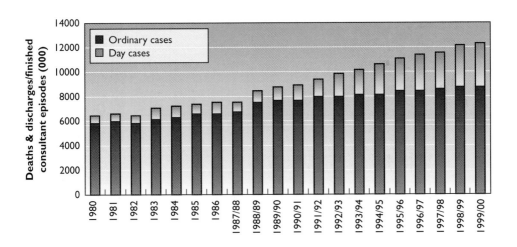

Accident and emergency activity: England

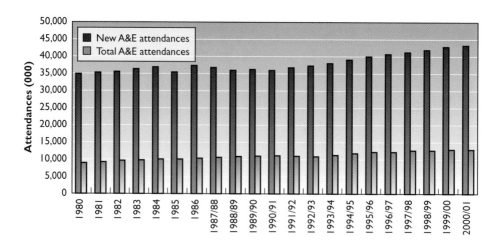

Outpatient activity: England

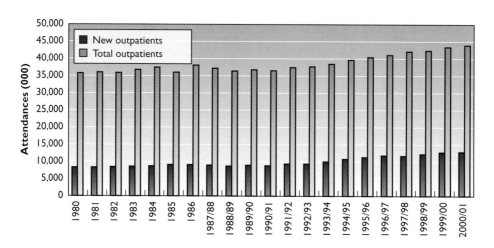

STAFF

Consultants: England

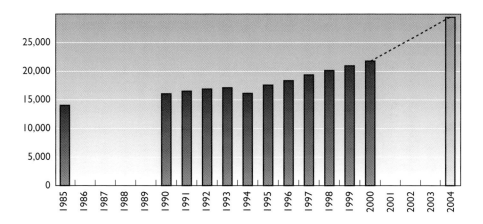

General practitioners: England

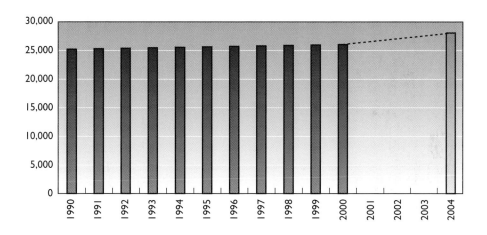

Hospital nurses and midwives: England

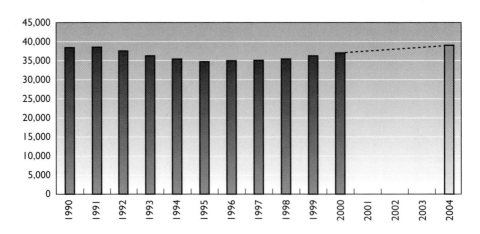